Evolution and Posttraumatic Stress

Posttraumatic stress disorder (PTSD) remains one of the most contentious and poorly understood psychiatric disorders. *Evolution and Posttraumatic Stress* provides a valuable new perspective on its nature and causes.

This book is the first to examine PTSD from an evolutionary perspective. Beginning with a review of conventional theories, Chris Cantor provides a clear and succinct overview of the history, clinical features and epidemiology of PTSD before going on to introduce and integrate evolutionary theory. Subjects discussed include:

- A clinical perspective of PTSD.
- The evolution of human defensive behaviours.
- Defence in overdrive – evolution, mammalian defences and PTSD.

This original presentation of PTSD as a defensive strategy describes how the use of evolutionary theory provides a more coherent and successful model for diagnosis and treatment, greatly improving understanding of usually mystifying symptoms. It will be of great interest to psychiatrists, psychologists, psychotherapists, sociologists and anthropologists.

Chris Cantor is Adjunct Senior Lecturer in Psychiatry at the University of Queensland, Australia.

Evolution and Posttraumatic Stress

Disorders of vigilance and defence

Chris Cantor

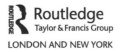
Routledge
Taylor & Francis Group

LONDON AND NEW YORK

First published 2005
by Routledge
27 Church Road, Hove, East Sussex BN3 2FA

Simultaneously published in the USA and Canada
by Routledge
711 Third Avenue, New York NY 10017

Routledge is an imprint of the Taylor & Francis Group

Copyright © 2005 Chris Cantor

Typeset in Times by RefineCatch Ltd., Bungay, Suffolk

Paperback cover design by Lou Page

British Library Cataloguing in Publication Data
A catalogue record for this book is available from the British Library

Library of Congress Cataloging-in-Publication Data
Cantor, Chris.
    Evolution and posttraumatic stress: disorders of vigilance and
defence / Chris Cantor.
        p.   cm.
    Includes bibliographical references and index.
    ISBN 1-58391-770-5 (hbk) – ISBN 1-58391-771-3 (pbk)
1. Post-traumatic stress disorder. 2. Evolutionary psychology.
    [DNLM: 1. Evolution. 2. Stress Disorders, Post-Traumatic.
3. Behavior, Animal. 4. Genetics, Behavioral. 5. Psychology,
Comparative.] I. Title.
    RC552.P67C36   2005
    616.85′21–dc22   2005001407

ISBN 978-1-58391-771-8 (pbk)

To Linda Mealey – thanks

Contents

Preface

> The truth is fairest naked, and the simpler its expression the profounder its influence.
>
> Arthur Schopenhauer, 1788–1860

Evolutionary theories of morphology are accepted by all medical practitioners, zoologists and virtually everyone else understanding human or animal anatomy. Aristotle's observations in marine biology circa 340 BC recognized that organisms might be related by descent, more than two millennia before Charles Darwin. Darwin (1871) merely proposed the means by which this occurs – natural and sexual selection, coevolution and the evolution of behaviour (Stearns and Hoekstra 2000).

Darwin offended his generation by suggesting there was no fundamental difference between humans and the higher mammals in their mental functions (Darwin 1871). Many researchers continue to be wary about evolution and behaviour. Why is this? Do mammals not all breathe in remarkably similar fashion? Is it not the case that all mammals reproduce by use of the seemingly primitive behaviour we call copulation? *Homo sapiens* may be a bit more romantic about it, but this very peculiar behaviour is the same fundamental equation across all mammalian, reptilian, avian, insectivorous and other species. Did these millions of species all discover this peculiar pastime independently? Of course this behaviour is the product of evolution. Following on from this line of reasoning, can any individual or species survive long without defensive behaviour?

At its most simple level, the theory I propose is that posttraumatic stress disorder (PTSD), as well as being a psychological disorder, reflects defensive behaviours that have been adaptive in our ancestral past and have arisen via natural selection.

While some of the theories I suggest lend themselves to simple experimental design, they may be physically demanding. They require some brave souls to trudge through jungles of central Africa, evade civil wars, perhaps scale mountain slopes and avoid tropical diseases, just to name a few of the challenges. I looked around at some of my portly middle-aged colleagues in mental health and decided that even if some of them were mad enough to agree my ideas had merit, how many were up to the physical challenge? Primatologists and anthropologists seemed a more likely lot. That meant a need to familiarize them with what is known about PTSD.

Some of my ideas do not require such field-testing; they can be explored in clinics by the portly and advanced in years. However, mostly I am referring to veterinary clinics. Who is more likely to be awarded a major research grant to study traumatized animals – a psychiatrist, psychologist or a vet? I talked to a few leading veterinary researchers familiar with animal trauma; 'PTSD? What is that?' appeared the response.

So my audience needed to include all types of mental health practitioners and researchers, veterinarians, zoologists, anthropologists, primatologists, sociologists and various others. How many of them would read psychiatric journals or complex psychiatric texts? If this work is to stimulate researchers to venture into places like the remoter regions of central Africa and other locations where psychiatric clinics do not exist, but our great ape relatives are to be found, an accessible style of writing was required.

This book is about proposing new theories, largely by way of crossing multiple disciplines. It does not try to provide comprehensive coverage from each disciplinary perspective. If it did, it would be well over a thousand pages long, no publisher would touch it and hardly anyone would want to wade through it. The coverage of particular research areas needs only to be sufficient to provide a basis for the ideas I propose. Those wanting more in-depth coverage should turn to the references cited. To cater for diverse readers, I will limit the unnecessary use of technical terms. However, I have included a glossary of technical terms, which I encourage readers in unfamiliar territory to use.

> All truth passes through three stages. First, it is ridiculed. Second, it is violently opposed. Third, it is accepted as self-evident.
> Arthur Schopenhauer, 1788–1860

Acknowledgements

Where does one start with trying to write such a book as this? Where others have left off is usual. However, literature searches revealed nothing substantial. Although it seemed difficult to believe, the topic of evolution and PTSD had been overlooked. I struggled with the task of laying foundations from scratch and wrote to experts in various disciplines. Eventually, suggestions gave rise to coherence and what began as a trickle of ideas became a flowing stream.

I thank those who helped with these inquiries including: Robert Atkinson, Gordon Burghardt, Cam Day, Ross Eastgate, Sue Gallagher, Russell Gardner, Melissa Lindeman, Isaac Marks, Susan Mineka, Helen Munro, Fran Norris, Craig Packer, Samantha Scott, Mike Speed, Adrian Treves, Clifford Warwick and Richard Wrangham. A special thanks goes to my patients for sharing their experiences with me and teaching me so much. I also thank the University of Queensland and its librarians for their helping me find research materials.

This book benefited greatly from helpful comments on early drafts from the following colleagues and friends: Geoff Acton, Becky Cantor, Russell Gardner, Jerry Gelb, Paul Gilbert, Ivor Jones, Alexander McFarlane, John Price and Tina Sweeney. Russell deserves a special encore as his generosity with time was extreme.

Finally, my undying gratitude goes to my original mentor in evolutionary studies, Linda Mealey, whose work and encouragement served as an early inspiration to me. Linda tragically died of cancer, before I had completed the first draft of this book. I hope that her enthusiasm was not wasted on me.

Chris Cantor
University of Queensland

Introduction

Increasingly, psychological disorders are being revisited from evolutionary perspectives (Stevens and Price 1996). For those new to reconceptualizing illness in evolutionary perspectives, a few cautions are needed. Darwin did not view evolution as following any predetermined design or direction – there is no end goal (Birx 1997). Darwin had misgivings about the term 'evolution' because of its potential to be misinterpreted. Evolution is neither static nor without error. The environmental background on earth has been, and will be, forever changing until the planet meets its eventual demise, let us hope in the distant future.

We live in a most remarkable age of civilization, quite unlike that for which most of our genes evolved. Mostly, PTSD in this twenty-first century will be maladaptive – a case of wrong time and place. If a psychological disorder is maladaptive, why would it persist? The key answer I believe is that a small dose of PTSD may have been highly adaptive, but a large one less so. Being tall may seem an advantage for males, but beyond a certain point it quickly becomes a liability. Other answers to this question include the following (McGuire et al. 1992). Deviant traits usually reduce evolutionary fitness, as opposed to preclude it, hence, it takes time for maladaptive traits to disappear. Many disorders emerge in the lifespan after peak reproduction periods – for example, Alzheimer's disease. Organisms with mixed genes for a particular characteristic may be fitter than those with identical genes – this is known as 'heterosis' and an example is the condition sickle cell anaemia, in which an entire set of similar (homozygous) deviant genes may be fatal, but carrying mixed (heterozygous) genes for it may be beneficial, by enhancing resistance to malaria. Recessive traits may be difficult to eliminate if they only partially compromise adaptation. Some behaviours that are maladaptive in some cultures may not be in others – for example, attention deficit hyperactivity disorder may seem disadvantageous in our orderly modern world, but would have been less so in times more compatible with chaotic youngsters. Lastly, some so-called 'pathology' may in fact be adaptive – suppressing fever with anti-pyretic medications may prolong some infections and similarly low plasma iron levels may deprive bacteria of vital minerals, hence iron supplements in some infections may also be counterproductive (Williams and Nesse 1991).

Often evolution involves costs of a surprising magnitude (Nesse and Williams 1998). Trade-offs are widespread. In humans the benefits of infants being born with large brains, that at times are incom-patible with the size of the female birth canal, have been associated with millions or even billions of mothers dying in childbirth (Gilbert 1998).

The structure of the book

After these introductory remarks, I will now orientate readers to what follows. Part I is a basic overview of PTSD. I will review the history and contemporary clinical understanding of PTSD, before examining conventional theories of causation. In the process I will emphasize animal research as no evolutionary work could do other-wise. I also use case histories from my clinical practice to illustrate issues. I have deliberately disguised some of these to protect con-fidentiality. Part II travels back to the beginning of life and from there traces the evolution of defence. I then put it all together, proposing many new theories and ideas – some broad, others specific; some highly probable, others considerably less so. Hypotheses emerge, some of which will be surprisingly easy to test experimentally.

Chapter 1 provides a brief history of the study of trauma, espe-cially as it relates to the recent arrival of PTSD as a conceptual entity. Chapter 2 presents an overview of PTSD as a clinical dis-order. It outlines what traumas and symptoms are currently accepted as being involved. It discusses some variants to its stereotypic presen-tation. It describes briefly risk factors and epidemiology. Chapter 3 examines the three dominant conventional aetiological theories of PTSD including the political contexts in which they have emerged.

In Chapter 4 I return to the beginning of life and trace our ances-tral journey from its earliest origins to the present day. I review our ancestry from the perspective of defences, emphasizing the reptilian and mammalian eras and their influences on our contemporary genetic make-up. Humans, like other animals, are individuals living in contexts. Predation and foraging cost–benefit equations add complexity to individual perspectives on defence. I review the likely defensive strategies of the pre-hominid and hominid eras, albeit with help from research on contemporary species.

Thereafter, it is crunch time. I apply the evolutionary theories to existing knowledge about PTSD. Some conclusions I suggest wear the cloak of near certainty; others are obviously speculative. Chapter 5 outlines the evolutionary theory of PTSD, linking it with clinical symptomatology. Chapters 6 to 9 revisit the mammalian defences introduced in Chapter 4, all of which are dependent on vigilance and risk assessment. All six of these defences are to be found by those working with traumatized persons if they are familiar with what to look for. Chapter 10 addresses the classic question of PTSD research, namely why some trauma victims but not others develop the condition. It suggests new answers and emphasizes the need for closer attention to the context of traumas. It concludes with a succinct summation of the fully assembled theory. The epilogue constitutes both an appeal and guidance to veterinarians, anthropologists, primatologists and other animal workers to consider these issues in domesticated and wild animals.

Part I

Posttraumatic stress disorder

An introduction

We rarely think people have good sense unless they agree with us.
François de la Rouchefoucauld, 1613–1680

Chapter 1

A brief history of PTSD

> When a thing ceases to be a subject of controversy, it ceases to be a subject of interest.
>
> William Hazlitt, 1778–1830

The long and the short

Posttraumatic stress disorder was once thought to be relatively uncommon, but recent estimates suggest that between 10 and 39 per cent of people will suffer it during their lives (Breslau et al. 1998; Kilpatrick and Resnick 1992). For many the disorder becomes chronic and disabling. In 2002 a class action suit was brought by 2000 British service personnel against the UK Ministry of Defence relating to psychological trauma sustained in conflicts including Northern Ireland, the Falklands, Bosnia and the first Gulf War. The action was largely unsuccessful, in part because of shortcomings in our factual base regarding psychological trauma prevention, but it nevertheless sounded a loud warning for the future (Bisson 2003). PTSD can no longer be ignored. In the search for knowledge there is a tendency to repeat research confirming what we already know, as opposed to probing new territory (McFarlane and van der Kolk 1996b). This book ventures into new territory. PTSD simply put is a complex and persistent reaction to severely threatening life experiences. It has an irrational or phobic quality, but unlike ordinary phobias it usually involves other elements, particularly a marked irritability or aggression. I will briefly describe two typical cases to orientate those unfamiliar with it.

An experienced policeman was called to a minor football match when the crowd of mainly intoxicated young adults became unruly. The rowdy contingent constituted over a hundred individuals. Prior experiences suggested that such youngsters generally settled down when diplomatically confronted. Unexpectedly, the policeman's partner was struck from behind. He went to his partner's aid and was himself struck from behind. He recalls being in a dazed state struggling with someone who was trying to remove his pistol from its holster. Eventually fourteen police officers brought the crowd under control. Subsequently, he struggled with the unexpectedness of what had transpired and his sense of powerlessness. He started shaking when called to domestic incidents. Two years later he has had to abandon his police career, he has difficulty sleeping, cannot cope with his anxiety in shopping centres, avoids watching television news because of its crime and war coverage, is highly socially reclusive, is irritable and particularly prone to automatically overreacting with uncharacteristic aggression to minor loutish behaviour in public, despite no longer carrying any policing responsibilities.

A government worker visited a remote rural household unaware of the householder's anti-government sentiments. She was confronted by the householder with a rifle in an obviously highly disturbed state of mind. She had no doubt that the householder meant to kill her. She compassionately identified with the householder's distress and her skilled negotiation of the situation probably saved her life. Subsequently, over several months she lost confidence in her work and eventually had to pursue medical retirement. Four years later, she remains socially avoidant and prone to fleeing from the few friends she does visit, if their voices become raised. She cannot sleep, is highly on edge when away from her home and is irritable. Minor day-to-day hassles become mountains for her. At interview she is recurrently overaroused and fragile, quite able to understand her abnormal reactions but relatively powerless to control them.

Having given you a taste of the condition, I need to make three key points regarding the history of PTSD. The first is how long it is; the second is how short it is; and the third is how blurred it is.

The early history of PTSD has been traced back to descriptions of trauma resembling PTSD in the pre-Christian period (Parry-Jones and Parry-Jones 1994). From the nineteenth century onwards a bewildering array of labels and concepts were described. These have included: 'spinal concussion', 'railway spins' and 'irritable heart' from the 1860s; 'soldier's heart' and 'cardiac weakness' from the 1870s; 'traumatic shock', 'traumatic neurosis', 'hysterical hemianaesthesia', 'spinal irritation', 'railway brain' and 'nervous shock' from the 1880s; 'anxiety neurosis' and 'psychical trauma' from the 1890s; 'traumatic neurosis', 'shell fever', 'irritable heart of soldiers', 'mental shock', 'war shock', 'shell shock', 'neuro-circulatory asthenia', 'disordered action of the heart' and 'war psychoneurosis' from the 1910s; 'cardiac/war neurosis' from the 1930s; and 'battle fatigue/combat exhaustion' and 'effort syndrome' from the 1940s (Parry-Jones and Parry-Jones 1994). Yet it was only as recently as 1980 that PTSD gained official recognition.

The above references to 'railways' relate to the early era of train travel, with one notable victim being the author Charles Dickens. When travelling by train, a crash had left his carriage swaying precariously from a bridge. On emerging, he saw dead and injured all around, but like a true professional went back to his carriage to get his manuscript. One year later Dickens noted, 'I have sudden vague rushes of terror, even when riding in a hansom cab, which are perfectly unreasonable but quite unsurmountable' (Beveridge 1997). His daughter suggested he never fully recovered. He died on the fifth anniversary of this train crash. Another British writer, Samuel Pepys, is also thought to have suffered PTSD, following the Great Fire of London in 1666. His subsequent irritability seems to have made him a boorish guest at London's celebrity dinners (Daly 1983).

The world wars

While railways heavily influenced the study of psychological trauma in the nineteenth century, wars were the dominant influences in the twentieth century. The First World War resulted in 80,000 British soldiers presenting with symptoms of 'shell shock' (Beveridge 1997). This embarrassed not only the military establishment but also British psychiatry, which until then had emphasized degeneracy and feeble minds. The fact that officers were five times more likely to develop psychiatric disorders than their fellow men helped reduce such bigotry and mobilize at least transient sympathy (Shephard 2002). However, in the years following the war the economic costs of unprecedented psychological casualties of war soon eroded the British government's sympathy. While the social intolerance of British veterans' 'weaknesses' was appalling (McFarlane and van der Kolk 1996a), in Germany it was even worse. Their fallen heroes were accused of being moral invalids not only for breaking down mentally but also for having failed to return victorious (van der Kolk et al. 1996b).

Generally psychiatry has had an ambivalent orientation with the notion that psychological trauma can profoundly and at times permanently alter brain functioning. Then and subsequently, there have been periods of fascination with and sympathy for those with PTSD, alternating with disbelief and condemnation (Shephard 2002).

Reviewing the contemporary descriptions of traumatic stress reactions is confusing as the accounts are through the eyes of writers of the time, there were no reliable research studies and the timing of presentations is confused. Acute stress reactions at the source of the stress – near the front lines – inevitably will be more dramatic than those removed from it, and from those months or years later. Hysteria, rightly or wrongly, was often diagnosed. This confuses but does not negate PTSD, as there is no reason why the two should not coexist. Accounts of bizarre motionless posturing suggestive of hysteria (these days called conversion or dissociative disorders) were common in both world wars (Shephard 2002).

Hysterical disorders have as a central characteristic the inability of individuals to face the sources of their traumas. While this is readily understandable in psychological terms, it is commonly encountered in the context of other medical or psychological illnesses, which often go overlooked. One of the 'medical' causes that would have fuelled hysterical reactions in the hideously long trench-warfare engagements of the First World War would have simply been exhaustion. This combined with artillery shelling and mortality on a scale never before experienced would have fuelled both hysterical and PTSD reactions. The futility of some battles, such as the Somme, would have massively added perceptions of uncontrollability and hopelessness to the soldiers' experiences. We will later see that uncontrollability is a particularly powerful inducer of anxiety states.

One lesson had seemed to have been learnt from the First World

War – that the cost of loss of fighting men by inappropriate psychological management was too great to ignore. Nevertheless, come the Second World War, it was disregarded. Winston Churchill, the British Prime Minister, was less than enamoured with the prospect of allowing psychiatrists and psychologists any chance of influencing the forthcoming torrent of casualties (Shephard 2002). The total annual cost of mental health services allocated to the British Army at that time has been estimated as the same as the cost of running the war for one hour and twenty minutes.

Whereas the First World War often involved lengthy immersion in the extreme horrors of the trenches, the Second World War generally meant briefer but at times more intense combat contacts, alternating with removal from the front line (Shephard 2002). This was most obvious in the air forces, where a pilot could wake up in relative comfort, spend the day flying while attempting to defy the high odds of being killed, to return from such hellish experiences to the comforts of home by the day's end.

Early conceptualization of traumatic reactions

The late nineteenth and early twentieth centuries were influenced by more notable writers in the field than I can describe in this short review, but brief orientation is desirable. 'Railroad spine' of the nineteenth century was emphatically 'organic' to some and 'psychological' to others, reflecting an unhealthy polarity of conceptualization that is slowly receding.

Pierre Janet, the French psychologist and neurologist, suggested that emotions may make events traumatic by interfering with the integration of experience into existing memory schemes. They are stored instead as anxiety phenomena or visual images that might resemble the emergency responses, but have little bearing on the current experience (van der Kolk 1994). Janet's work on the splitting or dissociation of conscious awareness of trauma in the early 1900s was quickly put to sleep for the middle part of the twentieth century, only to be rediscovered in the 1980s (van der Kolk et al. 1996b).

Sigmund Freud's work emphasized the destructive effects on the psyche of early sexual trauma (van der Kolk 1994). Although he expressed hope that neurophysiology would eventually explain many of his findings, his work at a time of primitive understanding of such issues contributed to the further separation of the mind from the brain.

Abram Kardiner (1941) more than anyone else in the middle twentieth century contributed positively to the limited progress of that era (van der Kolk et al. 1996b). Kardiner noticed the enduring vigilance of those suffering traumatic neuroses. He described this as a 'physioneurosis', a word that implied reuniting the physiological with the conflictual. His reconceptualization is highly relevant to the theories I later propose.

Science and politics in recent times

It would be nice if it could be said that mental health could have carried on from where Kardiner left off. However, the reality is that the former appeared to be in a state of scientific slumber. When the study of trauma finally reawakened it was due more to politics than scientific progress (Shephard 2002).

The influential American Psychiatric Association (APA) classificatory series known as the *Diagnostic and Statistical Manual(s) of Mental Disorders* (DSM) has both reflected and helped steer trauma-related psychiatry in the second half of the twentieth century. The first and second editions of the DSM series emphasized individual vulnerability with respect to trauma (Yehuda and McFarlane 1995). These early DSM editions had moved from feeble minds to neurotic ones. It was only in the third edition of the DSM series in 1980 (DSM-III) that PTSD gained official recognition, with a more balanced orientation (APA 1980). It would be tempting to think that psychiatry had become enlightened, but the acceptance of PTSD in the DSM-III was more about political lobbying than the wisdom of the profession. The Vietnam War had generated a band of advocates among the public who were not inclined to take 'no' for an answer (Shephard 2002).

While the DSM-III was a genuine milestone from both human rights and scientific perspectives, the phenomenologically symptom-based (as opposed to a basis in theory) orientation of the DSM series has decontextualized psychiatry. The multiple squabbling and divergent factions in mental health could not agree on causation of the many disorders, so the DSM largely banished causal factors from its diagnostic schemes. Agreement on symptom patterns was elevated to a far higher status than understanding what their underlying causes might be. Generally in medicine causation forms the basis of diagnostic classification. 'Chest disease' might have been acceptable as a diagnosis a few millennia ago. These days, specific subcategories based on causes such as tuberculosis, cancer, asthma, etc. are required. Mental health is yet to have the confidence necessary for consensuses on causation. Research was sorely needed and temporarily this seemingly bizarre atheoretical approach was probably justified. In time the DSM series will surely self-destruct or evolve into an aetiologically based system.

While causative factors are mostly banished from DSM diagnostic criteria, PTSD is one of the few disorders in which a partial causal attribution is recognized – i.e. massive trauma causing the problem. Nevertheless, an uneasy tension between those emphasizing trauma and those emphasizing individual vulnerability continues (van der Kolk and McFarlane 1996).

Within, between and beyond psychiatry, psychology and sociology there has been conflict between those wishing to normalize the status of victims and those wishing to define their states as abnormal (Yehuda and McFarlane 1995). Advocates of human rights and feminism have been reluctant to accept notions of damaged individuals, especially in the contexts of political oppression (for example, torture victims). This makes great political sense, provided one's priority is 'the Cause', as opposed to helping the suffering individuals. The fact that following most severe traumas, the majority of victims do not develop PTSD, suggests individual vulnerability, including genetic, familial, personality factors, past trauma problems and deficient supports. Achieving the correct balance between the responsibility of society and that of the individual is far from straightforward, especially when it comes to compensation.

Normality is often a confusing and unhelpful concept in mental health. In a statistical sense PTSD at times may emerge as 'normal' in the contexts of extreme traumas such as severe torture where the majority of those exposed may develop the disorder. With lesser stressors the same symptoms would be statistically 'abnormal'. Fortunately, in clinical practice it is all too obvious that PTSD is a psychological state associated with high levels of suffering and psychosocial disability. Many psychological disorders for which there is no controversy about 'normality', for example other anxiety disorders, may be less disabling. I suggest to patients that the debate about normal/abnormal mental health is frivolous. If their suffering is worth the effort of their consulting a mental health practitioner, it will be very rare that they would be wasting anyone's time. Ample stigma remains, deterring people from presenting for mental health care. Psychiatry is one of the last medical disciplines to recognize the benefits of early intervention. Even mild PTSD meets the threshold for legitimate health care need by a country mile.

There is one aspect of normality that I must strongly emphasize. PTSD is not a normal response to ordinary stressors. This is most important when considering results from animal experiments. There are ethical constraints on what mistreatments may be inflicted on animals for scientific purposes. Stressing them is permitted, but stressing them to the levels associated with PTSD generally is not. Hence, animal experiments at times confound the issue of normal stress responses and PTSD.

Muddy waters

A further confounding issue in the study of trauma is the blurring of boundaries between fear and loss-related phenomena. I will illustrate this with the most appalling and remarkable early case study I know of in the whole of mental health literature.

Parry-Jones and Parry-Jones (1994) described the observations of Dr Nicolai of Demonte and Professor Ignazio Somis.

The peasant family of Joseph Roccia were engulfed by an avalanche in the Italian Alps in 1755. Joseph Roccia (aged 50) and his son James (aged 15) saw their home engulfed by a huge avalanche, with Joseph's wife (aged 40), daughter (aged 11), son (aged 2) and sister-in-law (aged 24) within it. Thirty-seven days later Joseph's wife, daughter and sister-in-law were dug out alive, although his infant son was dead. They had been confined for over five weeks in a space said to be 6 by 4 by 2½ feet, within a hay manger partly protected by a beam. They had survived on a few chestnuts in one of their pockets, milk from two goats trapped with them, and snow. A donkey and two fowls died early in the drama. On the sixth day, Joseph's 2-year-old son was writhing in agony. Four days later he died in the arms of his distraught mother. The three remaining bereaved family members lived for three and a half weeks further, with the stench of the decomposing donkey, fowls, the little boy and their own faeces. In their final days of confinement, light heralded their coming rescue. However, according to folk beliefs of the time they interpreted the light as the death fires, believed to portend approaching death.

The two physicians Demonte and Somis conducted follow-up observations on the family from two days to two years after the tragedy. Joseph's wife could not leave her bed for six weeks and at three months was almost bald. She and the other two survivors had been helped during the ordeal by their submitting to their beliefs in the will of God. The other two survivors had suffered similar ordeals but apparently recovered within weeks with no obvious psychological problems. The traumatized and bereaved mother suffered insomnia, nightmares and intrusive recollections of the death of her son, was restricted to her home for two years before she could return to the fields, experienced an exaggerated startle reaction, suffered 'unconquerable watchfulness' and emotional lability and was generally disabled for more than two years (Parry-Jones and Parry-Jones 1994).

Mrs Roccia's symptoms were consistent with what we would now call PTSD. However, she was also thought to have suffered nutritional deficiencies and was probably depressed. One of the weakest aspects of PTSD is its blurred margins and tendency to coexist with other disorders. Comorbidity, the co-occurrence of other psychological or medical disorders, has been found in as many as 50–90 per cent of PTSD sufferers (Yehuda and McFarlane 1995). The key point I wish to make is that this early example of psychological trauma is decidedly muddy. Mrs Roccia had a horrific experience from the perspective of fear of her own surely certain and truly terrible lingering death. She had time to reflect on her loss and endured being trapped with her decomposing young son. She faced probable further bereavements, if she herself did not die next. Her physical health was also compromised. The sight of death is never pretty, but this combination of insults over such a period must have provoked horror and revulsion on a scale rarely experienced.

The neuroscience of fear, loss, disgust and medical illness is likely to involve different physiological processes mediating such experiences. The experience of trauma frequently involves the co-occurrence of extreme fear and extreme loss. The study of responses to extreme fear, I suggest, involves PTSD; that of loss involves depression. Nowadays, if a person escapes a horrific car accident physically unscathed, PTSD may yet result. If loss is added to the equation, depression may ensue. Such loss may arise by way of the death of or serious injury to a significant other, loss of function (and often income) due to physical or psychological injury, or even as a result of the justice system whose wheels of motion may take an eternity to clear a driver of criminal negligence. Pure PTSD does exist. However, the confounding effects of loss and depression have all too often blurred the study of PTSD.

Historically, the study of trauma in psychiatry started from an undifferentiated state. Horrific events are traumatic, regardless of their type. While all trauma is painful, we need to define the characteristics of trauma subtypes including anxiety, fear, loss, guilt, shame, revulsion and other painful emotions.

Early ethological speculations

The final area of history I will mention is that of the few studies that come closest to directly addressing the subject of this book. Ethology is the science of animal behaviour, which recognizes the centrality of evolution in any biological science. As early as 1953, Scott and Marston (1953) speculated that study of fighting behaviour in mice might provide some insights into 'combat fatigue'. Defeated mice were found to develop a persistent inhibition of fighting and persistent escape behaviour. Not too dissimilar from veterans of numerous wars. Almost half a century later, Derek Silove (1998) may have been the first to publish a paper specifically on the evolutionary aspects of PTSD. Isaac Marks (1987) in an exemplary text had previously traced the development of withdrawal behaviours from the single celled protozoa through to humans, yet had relatively little to say about PTSD, perhaps reflecting the short history at the time of PTSD as an official entity. Ohman et al. (1985) suggested that phobias provide examples of biologically prepared learned responses that were once relevant to humans' ancestors. Again at that time PTSD was still in its infancy. Nesse (1997) has presented an evolutionary perspective on panic disorder and agoraphobia. Stevens and Price (1996) have written a text *Evolutionary Psychiatry*, but such an all-embracing and pioneering work inevitably could not approach PTSD in any depth. The evolution of PTSD to date has essentially been overlooked.

Literature searches and my speaking directly to several leading veterinary researchers seem to suggest that while psychiatrists have been tardy accepting the legitimacy of PTSD as a concept, veterinarians have barely crossed the starting line. One text, *Psychopharmacology of Animal Behavior Disorders*, accepts and uses the DSM-IV human psychopathology model (Dodman and Shuster 1998). It does note some reservations: first, vets are more accustomed to using objective as opposed to the more subjective data of the DSM-IV; second, I quote: 'given the importance of evolutionary and ethologic theory in comparative biology, a comparative clinical psychopharmacology might immediately move toward classification systems that rely on these theories' (Stein 1998). The author is saying, in effect, that one of the shortcomings of the DSM-IV is its neglect of evolutionary considerations. Nevertheless, in the absence of an alternative comprehensive classificatory scheme for abnormal animal behaviour, the DSM-IV system prevailed. An important and perhaps surprising point is that this text suggests that there is little reason to believe that animal psychopathology does not broadly parallel human psychopathology. Scientists with a compassionate orientation to animals may have been able to identify with their suffering; others orientated to the suffering of fellow humans may have remained too aloof to notice the similarities. Pet owners have never had such problems.

Although data are not presented, Dodman and Shuster's (1998) veterinary text accepts that PTSD may arise in animals hit by motor vehicles, abused by strangers or unscrupulous individuals, stung by insects, or traumatized by fearful and poorly understood noises (Thompson 1998). Informal dialogue I have had with an experienced defence service dog handler suggested his familiarity with the notion of long-term anxious and aggressive responses in severely traumatized dogs. The detection of PTSD is greatly facilitated by subjective verbal accounts. If mental health practitioners can overlook the disorder up to 1980 (and some beyond) surely we can be gracious to our veterinary colleagues whose patients do not talk and have minimal capacity for abstract reasoning.

I suggest that an understanding of defence strategies in animals and humans provides remarkable insights into phenomena clinically encountered in those suffering PTSD. As veterinarians take up the mantle of PTSD, their own research should prove highly illuminating for those of us struggling to understand the disorder in humans.

Summary

There is evidence that PTSD is likely to have existed in much earlier times. It has been common in the history of psychiatry for belatedly recognized phenomena to be considered novel in origin – as opposed to overlooked. It is highly probable that the colours of PTSD reflect contemporary issues, but its essence is likely to be much older. Explorations in this area may be hindered if the separation of danger and loss-related phenomena is neglected. All animals are strongly responsive to danger. The more social ones, including ourselves, are also strongly responsive to loss.

Chapter 2

A clinical perspective of PTSD

Truth is beautiful, without doubt; but so are lies.
Ralph Waldo Emerson, 1803–1882

PTSD as a concept

In this chapter I need to introduce PTSD more formally to those unfamiliar with it and review its essentials for those readers already well acquainted with it. I will summarize the clinical and demographic details of PTSD that will be relevant for subsequent evolutionary considerations.

Trauma may produce a range of psychological reactions including depression, alcohol and drug abuse, PTSD and specific phobias. The generalized distress of PTSD is profoundly important for differentiating it from other phobic reactions. Even war veterans commonly are unable to visit shopping centres as if the enemy were likely to be there. Specific symptoms differentiating PTSD from other traumatic disorders include enduring exaggerated startle responses, hypervigilance and irritability (McFarlane and Yehuda 1996).

At the time of writing, the two dominant classificatory systems were the *International Statistical Classification of Diseases* (ICD-10) (World Health Organization [WHO] 1992) and the *Diagnostic and Statistical Manual of Mental Disorders* (fourth edition) (DSM-IV) (APA 1994). The publication of DSM-IV in 1994 involved criteria revisions following its predecessor, the DSM-III-R. I will use the DSM-IV as opposed to ICD-10 criteria, as the former are more explicit, although the two mostly are in accord with each other. One difference is that the DSM-IV lists PTSD as an anxiety disorder, whereas the ICD-10 grants it autonomous status.

Both the ICD-10 and DSM-IV agree that the consideration of

traumatic stress reactions should separate the early reaction (acute stress disorder) of the first month from the longer subsequent reaction. Despite the support for the concept of an acute stress disorder I will deliberately gloss over it, as there remains much uncertainty about its characteristics.

American psychiatry emphasizes the importance of dissociation as distinct from anxiety. Dissociation involves separation of mental or behavioural processes from the sense of self, for example 'the gun was pointed at me, but it was like I was not there; as if I was in a movie'. It involves a split between one's 'observing self' and one's 'experiencing self' (van der Kolk 1996a). Symptoms include numbing, reduced emotional responsiveness, reduced awareness of surroundings, feelings of unreality and psychogenic amnesia. Two major objections to conceptualizing PTSD as a dissociative disorder include the imprecision as to what exactly constitutes dissociation, particularly its boundaries, and the many dissimilarities between PTSD and the dissociative disorders (Brett 1996).

ICD-10 also provides for a more diffuse long-term reaction called 'Enduring personality changes after catastrophic experience' (Brett 1996), which approximates other terms 'complex PTSD' and 'DESNOS', both of which I will mention shortly.

The DSM-IV criteria for PTSD

PTSD as described in the DSM-IV is triggered by experiencing, witnessing or being confronted with an event or events that involve actual or threatened death or serious injury, or a threat to the physical integrity of self or others. In addition the person's response must involve intense fear, helplessness or horror (APA 1994). This definition of stressors represents a lowering of the threshold from earlier definitions, which emphasized the stressors as being those that would cause marked distress to almost anyone. Also, the earlier emphasis was on abnormal stressors impacting on normal personalities. This has been modified so that persons with vulnerable personalities can be accommodated. If major stressors can traumatize resilient individuals, why should less resilient persons be immune? There are complex conceptual problems with stressor definitions of great medico-legal importance (Tennant 2004). I do not want to get bogged down on the details, so will simply suggest that a clearer focus on defensive as opposed to loss reactions may aid progress, and then move on.

The DSM-IV requires symptoms from three clusters:

- Cluster B – re-experiencing phenomena (five items; one or more required for the diagnosis)
- Cluster C – avoidance behaviours (seven items; three or more required)
- Cluster D – overarousal symptoms (five items; two or more required).

Re-experiencing phenomena (briefly stated) include intrusive recollections such as images, thoughts, perceptions, etc. (item B1) and nightmares (B2) of the traumatic experiences. Acting or feeling as if the trauma was recurring (B3) may include a sense of reliving the experience, illusions, hallucinations and dissociative flashbacks.

> For example, a Vietnam War veteran had the unpleasant task of handling many bodies, which leaked body fluids and were decomposing in the tropical heat. More than thirty years later, he still regularly re-experiences the smell and even the taste of the bodies. He uses a handkerchief doused with his wife's perfume to mask these sensations.

The remaining DSM-IV re-experiencing items are intense psychological distress (B4) and physiological reactions (B5), both in response to reminders of the events. Television is a scourge to many PTSD sufferers with respect to these two items. Road safety advertisements designed to shock, by way of graphic accident portrayals, do more than shock viewers suffering motor vehicle accident induced PTSD.

Avoidance behaviours include avoiding thoughts, feelings or conversations associated with the trauma (item C1); efforts to avoid activities, places or people arousing such recollections (C2); inability to recall an important aspect of the trauma (as if the mind has blanked it out) (C3); markedly diminished interest or participation in significant activities (C4); emotional detachment from (C5) and restricted feelings for other people (C6); and a sense of a foreshortened future (C7).

Overarousal symptoms include reduced hours of sleep (item D1); irritability/anger (D2); difficulty concentrating (D3); hypervigilance or feeling on edge in a number of situations (D4); and exaggerated startle responses (D5).

Another Vietnam veteran patient of mine has a hearing problem, as do so many who have experienced war in the front line. In public, if some innocent shopper happens to creep up on him unheard and unseen, he tends to instantly jump into an attack posture, only then to have to contain his fright while attempting to reassure the equally startled shopper.

De Bellis (2001) has suggested that re-experiencing phenomena can be best conceptualized as classically conditioned responses, avoidance behaviours as ways to control the pain of re-experiencing symptoms, and overarousal symptoms as dysregulation of the limbic hypothalamo-pituitary adrenal axis (a neuro-endocrine system). While there may be some truth in these suggestions, they involve switching models of understanding, from the psychological to the biological, to explain the phenomena, without a unifying theme. The model that I will develop integrates psychological and biological understandings. They are one and the same.

Biphasic alternation between intrusive re-experiencing phenomena and numbing avoidance phenomena may be a hallmark of PTSD (Horowitz 1986; van der Kolk 1987). Put simply, a sufferer's mind may alternate between feeling overwhelmed by traumatic memories and 'underwhelmed' by present-day experiences. They may be unable to forget their traumas, but extremely forgetful for everyday chores.

Foa et al. (1992) have suggested that the DSM-IV avoidance behaviours category can be subdivided into active avoidance of trauma-related thoughts or situations, and a more passive numbing of emotional responsiveness, including a restricted range of affect (mood), detachment and decreased interest in activities. The evolutionary theory discussed later will strongly support this suggestion. It has also been suggested that numbing (avoidance criteria C4, C5 and C6) may represent problems in expressive behaviour, felt emotion or both (Litz and Gray 2002). PTSD patients sometimes report choosing to withhold emotions as well as restricted feelings. Litz and Gray (2002) have suggested that the evidence does not support behavioural models that attribute numbing to chronic avoidance behaviours. Later, I will expand on this when we will find that experimentally traumatized mice have been reliably found to have numb tails – tails being convenient targets for inflicting pain. It would be difficult indeed to conceptualize numb tails as avoidance behaviours.

The nature of traumas and frequency of PTSD

PTSD is not simply a product of stress. By definition both the stressor and its result are unusually severe. What else characterizes the stressors? McFarlane and Girolamo (1996) suggest, 'Central to the experience of traumatic stress are the dimensions of helplessness, powerlessness, and threat to one's life. Trauma attacks the individual's sense of self and predictability of the world'. A wide variety of stressful experiences have been associated with PTSD including injury, violent or unexpected bereavement, witnessing or participating in abusive violence, exposure to grotesque death, hearing about the death of another person, life threat, rape, torture (Green 1994) and body handling (Deahl 2000).

People who have suffered torture and/or prolonged victimization understandably suffer the highest rates of PTSD. Prisoners of war and concentration camp survivors may have rates of chronic PTSD around 50 per cent, while survivors of natural disasters may have rates around 4 per cent (Yehuda et al. 1998). In another study, of ten traumatic events examined, tragic death was the most frequent trauma experienced, but sexual assault yielded the highest rates of PTSD (Norris 1992). Motor vehicle accidents presented the most adverse combination of frequency and impact with a lifetime prevalence of serious motor vehicle accidents of 23 per cent, with 12 per cent of those developing PTSD. The current (as opposed to lifetime) prevalence of PTSD in those exposed to violent crimes, tragic deaths or accidents was found to be 7–11 per cent as compared with 5–8 per cent of those exposed to environmental hazards.

Kushner et al. (1992) reviewed PTSD studies and suggested that about 50 per cent of rape victims and 30 per cent of non-sexual assault victims will develop PTSD within three months. Severity, type and duration of the rape contributed only a small proportion of the variance. Individual differences in victims appeared to play a role. Females experience non-sexual assault less frequently than males but have much higher rates of PTSD per assault (Breslau et al. 1999). It is likely that the greater expectations of, familiarity with and capacity to handle violence of males may be protective. Perception has great capacity to mediate traumatic experiences. Nevertheless, the magnitude of stressor exposure, previous trauma and lack of social support are the three most significant external predictors of chronic PTSD (van der Kolk 1994).

In more recent studies with better methodology, PTSD is increasingly being recognized as a common condition, with an influential study suggesting that 18 per cent of women and 10 per cent of men in the United States will develop PTSD (Breslau et al. 1998). Males generally are exposed to more traumatic events than women. Males are notorious risk-takers and even now are the dominant front-line victims of warfare. Younger age at the time of service was associated with greater risk of PTSD in Vietnam War combat veterans (Green et al. 1990). However, females seem to be more vulnerable to specific traumatic events. A study of 1500 women found lifetime prevalence rates of PTSD ranging from 10 to 39 per cent, with current rates ranging from 1 to 13 per cent (Kilpatrick and Resnick 1992).

Pooled results from a number of studies suggested that one-quarter of individuals exposed to DSM-IV criterion A stressor events (i.e. those of a sufficient magnitude to generate risk of PTSD) develop PTSD (Green 1994). An important implication of this finding is its inverse result – three-quarters of those experiencing such events do not develop PTSD. One of the most important research areas in this field is the tantalizing question of 'Why?' Perception may be one important explanation, but there is much more that remains a mystery. Some new suggestions will be provided in Chapter 10.

The influence of perception

Apparently trivial stressors sometimes may trigger PTSD in individuals because of the meaning attached to them. Consider a non-life-threatening injury such as losing a little finger. Competitive motorcyclists view crushing, losing or otherwise destroying their little fingers as an occupational hazard. Sooner or later one of their tumbles is going to find a little finger between the handlebars and the tarmac. Compare this with a concert pianist who is attacked and has his or her hand held down with a finger crushed maliciously by a hammer wielded by an intruder. Loss has potential to confound this example, but loss alone produces depression without PTSD. Research has found that where physical injury is incurred, *perceived* loss of function is more important than the extent of injury. Adequate preparation for the stressful event protects individuals from the effect of the stress (cf. motorcycle racers). It reduces uncertainty and increases one's sense of control (Shalev 1996). Similarly all medical doctors witness massive trauma in their hospital careers, yet to date I have not seen one with PTSD. The consideration of severity of stressor must include the consideration of perception.

A retired detective I saw developed PTSD following a pedestrian accident. He misjudged crossing the road as a bus made a sharp turn oblivious of him. His ankle twisted at just the wrong moment and he appeared likely to fall under the rear wheels of the bus. He expected to die, but fortunately bounced off, falling clear with only moderate physical injuries. His life history included the following: at age 6 a teacher in jest lunged at him with a bayonet terrifying him, leaving him with a lifelong disdain for teachers. In his twenties he was alarmed at the strength of his reaction to a criminal who lunged at him with a knife, though he managed to contain himself in subsequent similar incidents. He attended numerous murders, one of which involved a teacher who shot his wife. He was distressed by this and cleaned up the blood in the house prior to relatives arriving, although this was not part of his duties. He had extensive contact with the underworld, dealing with this by a sense of invincibility shared with his colleagues. He was able to laugh off the dangers and gruesome murders of underworld figures. He even felt invincible when a serious contract was taken out on his life. But it was the bus that penetrated his defences most. That and to a lesser extent the bayonet through the eyes of a youngster were the incidents he perceived as most distressing. No one writing his life history would have predicted that these two incidents would affect him the most. Perception is very personal.

A lower risk for PTSD has been found in those briefly unconscious following motor vehicle accidents (Mayou et al. 1993). This further supports the suggestion that perception of horror, in addition to threat to life, is part of the causation (Foa and Kozac 1986). This raises the intriguing possibility that administering amnesia-promoting drugs soon after discrete serious trauma might have a preventative role. PTSD may relate not so much to the severity of the stress response, but how it is processed (McFarlane 1997).

The World Trade Center, September 11 2001 terrorist attacks, in which over 3000 people died, are still being evaluated. However, a random phone survey of Manhattan residents five to eight weeks later suggested a diagnosis of PTSD in 7.5 per cent of 1008 adults surveyed (Galea et al. 2002a). The prevalence rose to 20 per cent among those living closer to the disaster site. As would be expected PTSD was higher in those more directly involved, e.g. those physically injured (30 per cent) (Galea et al. 2003). However, those indirectly exposed through repeatedly viewing television coverage of people falling from the World Trade Center were found to have high rates of PTSD if they were directly affected by the attacks (e.g. losing friends) (Ahern et al. 2002).

Generally stressors associated with crime or malice are associated with greater risk for PTSD (Yehuda and McFarlane 1995). Malice combined with the massive scale of the unpredicted and uncontrolled trauma of the World Trade Center events of September 11 2001 in New York and the October 2002 Balinese night-club bombing may be expected to result in high PTSD rates in survivors, witnesses, families, helpers and others less directly affected. At time of writing, the December 2004 South East Asian tsunami had recently occurred. This might be expected to produce lower rates of PTSD, when compared with a manmade catastrophe of a similar magnitude, such as a nuclear holocaust.

Trauma and symptom course

The type of trauma may relate to the subsequent course of PTSD. However, in the acute aftermath it is not possible to reliably predict who will develop PTSD, although some risk factors are recognized. Perhaps surprisingly, circumscribed traumas such as accidents may have more enduring effects than combat (McFarlane 1997). This may relate to both perceptions (discussed above) and predictability and controllability, which are explored in Chapter 3. War is expected to be nasty, though often such expectations prove well short of the mark. Accidents tend to catch people unawares, unless they are racing drivers, jockeys or such like who seem to survive psychologically to race on.

In a study of 188 motor vehicle accident victims, 18 per cent of individuals were found to have experienced an acute distress syndrome (Mayou et al. 1993). Only 15 per cent of the total had no problems at one year. Thirteen individuals had mood disorders, thirteen travel phobias but only nine suffered PTSD. PTSD is particularly likely to be chronic if it is accompanied by another comorbid anxiety disorder such as a travel phobia following a vehicle accident (Zlotnick et al. 1999).

Most remissions of PTSD occur in the first year in about 60 per cent of cases. If PTSD has not resolved within six years it is highly likely to remain chronic. Persistent dissociation in the early stress response is a predictor of later PTSD (Murray et al. 2002).

Paradoxically, some individuals with PTSD who may be irrationally preoccupied with safety are at risk of revictimization (McFarlane and van der Kolk 1996a). A battered spouse may leave her partner only to choose a partner others might recognize as a bad risk. Rape victims tend to be at risk of being raped again. Women and men sexually abused as children often may again be sexually abused as adults. Overt self-destructive behaviour is especially common with complex PTSD. This may involve self-mutilation, drug abuse and eating disorders.

War studies

The combination of the novelty of both the concept of PTSD and appropriate research methods unfortunately limit any meaningful comparison of the Vietnam War with earlier major wars, especially the First and Second World Wars. Some might expect the appallingly high mortality and extreme conditions of many First World War battles to produce in turn extreme rates of PTSD, if it had been available as a concept to study at the time. A survey of over 300 Second World War veterans in a medical outpatient clinic of a Veterans Administration hospital was conducted by van der Kolk in 1982 (McFarlane and van der Kolk 1996a); 85 per cent of the clinic attendees were found to have suffered PTSD, but not one had any psychiatric diagnosis noted in their medical records.

The Vietnam War has dominated PTSD research as we struggle to make up for lost time. It has been estimated that 16 to 35 per cent of the 2.8 million Americans who served in Vietnam have suffered significant psychological problems (including but not confined to PTSD) as a result of combat exposure. This figure did not take into account those in prison, those currently hospitalized or those living in inaccessible areas (Egendorf et al. 1981). In another study, lifetime rates of PTSD in male combat Vietnam veterans were found to be 31 per cent, with a current rate of 15 per cent nineteen years after their combat experience. Acute distress experienced at combat was found to be proportional to subsequent PTSD symptoms, as might be expected (Kulka et al. 1990).

The Vietnam War may not have had as high mortality rates as the First and Second World Wars but some aspects of it might have generated disproportionate psychological trauma. The war was characterized by an unusual difficulty in identifying the enemy. In the dense jungle, enemy foot soldiers might be heard before they were seen. At times they were even smelt first, often being invisible to the enemy who might be only tens of yards away. Also, the sounds of gunshots and muzzle flashes made those firing weapons easier targets for the enemy to zero in on. The Americans and their allies fought alongside the South Vietnamese, who were of the same appearance as the North Vietnamese enemy. The Viet Cong infiltrated the south and were a serious threat, but often difficult to identify. Many innocent civilians were shot by soldiers fearing they were Viet Cong. Learning they were not was highly distressing, especially if they were female.

Wars, especially the Vietnam War, have contributed disproportionately to the research literature on PTSD. It can legitimately be asked whether such war experiences, which usually involve some expectation and preparation for traumas (plural) experienced over extended periods, produce the same reactions as, for example, a single traumatic peacetime accident.

Complex PTSD

'Complex PTSD' refers to a more complicated picture that may emerge when trauma occurs sufficiently early in a person's life, and/or over a sufficiently long duration, to affect his/her developmental course. Judith Herman (1992), an influential writer on the topic, pointed out that prolonged repeated trauma can occur in victims in states of 'captivity', when they are unable to flee and are under the control of their perpetrators. They may include physically and sexually abused children, battered wives and concentration camp survivors. Captives may use voluntary dissociation including the induction of trances to cope with torture.

Sexual abuse may be associated with shame, dissociation and effects on cultural constructions of self versus others. Abused children often use dissociation extensively, in part to cope with the trauma and in part to preserve the illusion of good parents. The results include characteristic personality changes, involving vulnerability to repeated harm inflicted by themselves and others, as seen in borderline personality and the rarer dissociative identity (multiple personality) disorders, both of which often display post-traumatic stress elements. Herman (1992) emphasized somatic, dissociative and affective (mood) sequelae. Loss of identity may occur.

> One such patient has recurrently protested to me: 'I am not a person; I am an IT!' After several years in treatment she still resented my addressing her by her name. She recently officially changed it and I find it incredibly difficult to reliably use her new name.

De Bellis (2001) has suggested that child maltreatment may be regarded as 'an environmentally induced complex developmental disorder'. Risk factors include: first, factors preceding the trauma – poor prior social support, adverse life events, parental poverty, prior maltreatment, poor family functioning, family history of psychiatric disorders, introversion or extreme behavioural inhibition, poor health and former mental illness; second, factors relating to the trauma – the degree of trauma exposure, chronicity of exposure and subjective responses; third, factors following the trauma – lack of support, continued negative life events (e.g. change of school or home), repeated threats, fear of the perpetrator of the abuse and financial disadvantage.

PTSD occurring in childhood may send the child's development along an abnormal trajectory. For example, fear and irritability may impact on peer relationships and disrupt educational achievements. Some children recurrently abused by their parents either are not allowed to bring friends home or are too afraid or embarrassed to do so. Roth et al. (1997) suggest that it remains unclear whether complex PTSD is qualitatively or quantitatively different from ordinary PTSD. My later reasoning in Chapter 8 strongly suggests a qualitative difference.

The DSM-IV panel considered introducing the label 'Disorders of Extreme Stress Not Otherwise Specified' (DESNOS) to cater for this. This rather pompous rubbish-basket label would have technically moved complex PTSD out of the way of ordinary PTSD, but would have dumped it in with miscellaneous other conditions. The DSM-IV did not proceed with this, but the alternative ICD-10 classification did include the explicit, if long label, 'Enduring personality changes after catastrophic experience' (Brett 1996). This includes permanent hostility and distrust, social withdrawal, feelings of emptiness and hopelessness, increased dependency, problems with modulation of aggression, hypervigilance, irritability, and feelings of alienation (van der Kolk 1996a).

Delayed PTSD

Patients not uncommonly present for treatment for the first time many years after their traumatic experiences. This phenomenon of delayed PTSD adds further complexity and controversy. The DSM-IV defines this as involving a delay of six months or more between the relevant trauma and the onset of the syndrome (APA 1994). In cases of civilian trauma it has been found to occur in only 4.4–6.2 per cent of PTSD cases (Bryant and Harvey 2002). In clinical practice delayed PTSD is more common, with veterans from the Vietnam War often presenting for the first time to this day.

True delayed PTSD probably is rare, and requires prospective studies to accurately differentiate it from the illusion of delay in presentation frequently involved in retrospective studies and clinical practice. Several explanations for apparent delay have been suggested (Scurfield 1985) including: immediate onset, followed by remission and later recurrence; a period of numbing followed by the onset of acute symptoms; a gradual progression of evolving symptoms over years; and a protracted asymptomatic state followed by a life stressor that triggers overt PTSD. It is only the latter that is true delayed PTSD. Other mechanisms include: the original trauma response being subthreshold for diagnosis, with symptoms increasing over time; reappraisals of trauma heightening subsequent perceptions of threats; and subsequent traumas compounding the initial stress reaction.

The reactivation of PTSD in later life of Second World War veterans has been reported in association with physical ill health, retirement, loneliness, comorbid psychiatric illness, anniversaries, service reunions, alcohol abuse and psychotropic drugs. It has also been suggested that hard work and other activity may previously have been adaptive defences albeit with emotional constriction (MacLeod 1994).

A Second World War veteran recently described to me his lifetime of successful career and social functioning, which he believed broke down as a result of other veterans reaching out to him with good intentions, but reactivating memories that he had been pushing to the back of his mind for over half a century.

Subthreshold PTSD

The phenomenon of subthreshold PTSD is of crucial importance to the later evolutionary consideration of PTSD. It is a PTSD-like presentation, the symptoms of which fall short of official criteria. Fran Norris (1992) estimated in one of her studies that if one fewer DSM-III-R avoidance criterion (for example, two instead of three avoidance behaviours) had been allowed, rates of diagnosed PTSD would have doubled or trebled. She commented, 'PTSD represents only the tip of the iceberg in terms of experienced distress'. Rape and sexual assault victims have been found to experience a more than 50 per cent decline in PTSD symptoms between two weeks and three months after the assaults (Valentiner et al. 1996). After the Oklahoma City bombing in 1995 in which 167 people died, transient PTSD symptoms of some type were near universal (North et al. 1999) suggesting that PTSD may lie at the extreme end of a continuous spectrum of trauma reactions.

The National Vietnam Veteran Readjustment Study suggested the need to define a posttraumatic syndrome in which the full PTSD criteria are not met (Kulka et al. 1990). In extreme trauma such as torture or concentration camp experiences, PTSD may not be particularly unusual – it may even be the norm, experienced by most individuals exposed to the trauma. This concept of normality in no way lessens the suffering and need for treatment. It is highly likely that PTSD symptoms lie on a continuum with less severe and possibly less generalized symptoms within the range of 'normality'. What is less clear is whether there is a gradual transition across the spectrum. Bend a branch and it flexes; bend it further and it may flex further or snap. Some neurochemical findings appear quite different in PTSD (McFarlane 1997).

Summary

PTSD may constitute a range of predominantly fear-related incapacitating reactions to severely threatening trauma. The core symptoms by convention are divided threefold into re-experiencing phenomena, avoidance behaviours and overarousal symptoms. Research increasingly suggests that PTSD is a common disorder. A wide range of traumas may cause PTSD. These range from a melee of war experiences, or complex child abuse affecting development, to relatively circumscribed, extremely threatening short-lived individual traumas. Perception may amplify or minimize reactions and produce unique perspectives. Trauma frequently induces depressive reactions, which I suggest are mostly loss-related phenomena as opposed to fear related. Uncertainties regarding diagnostic criteria and subtypes are extensive. The uncertainty as to whether PTSD exists on a continuum with 'normal' reactions is a particularly relevant issue with respect to evolutionary considerations.

Chapter 3

Conventional theories of PTSD

He that never changes his opinions, never corrects his mistakes, will never be wiser on the morrow than he is today.

Tyron Edwards, 1809–1894

In this chapter I briefly review the three major current models of PTSD. This book examines PTSD from an evolutionary perspective and so will draw heavily on animal research; where possible, primate research will be given priority over that involving other animals. Primates are close relations of *Homo sapiens*, therefore, their behaviours are more directly relevant than those of rats, dogs and other convenient laboratory subjects (Mineka 1987). Study of non-human primates has already yielded valuable insights into attachment disorders and depression in humans (e.g. Suomi 1991).

While these and most other models of PTSD make useful contributions to understanding PTSD, none offers a comprehensive view of the disorder (Lee and Turner 1997). Evolutionary psychological perspectives, as we will later see, shift the emphasis from the uniqueness of human psychological phenomena to what humans share with the rest of the animal kingdom (Ohman et al. 2000; Greene 1999). Evolutionary theories are distal in perspective. As such they have potential to integrate the more conventional proximal models. However, in response to reticence from the mainstream, there has been a tendency for apologetic approaches to the study of evolutionary functions of anxiety; i.e. that it is speculative and teleological, yet such hypotheses can and are tested like any others (Marks and Nesse 1997). But first, the proximal.

LEARNING, CONTROLLABILITY
AND PREDICTABILITY

I'm not afraid of storms, for I am learning how to sail my ship.
Louisa May Alcott, 1832–1888

Of rats and men

Most of the behavioural research relevant to PTSD stems from
conditioning studies of phobic behaviour, especially that relating to
uncontrollable and unpredictable situations. Foa et al. (1992) have
persuasively argued that disturbances in animals subjected to uncontrollable and unpredictable aversive events resemble PTSD symptoms and might serve as a suitable animal model. While some
symptoms are too subjective, e.g. flashbacks and intrusive recollections, most PTSD symptoms can be observed in animals, including
distress on re-exposure to trauma stimuli, central to re-experiencing,
the most subjective of the three symptom clusters. Many of the
avoidance behaviours are flight or numbness orientated and so lend
themselves well to direct or physiological observations. Overarousal
symptoms other than memory problems are also readily observable
in animals. However, phobias differ from PTSD by not having
irritability as a core symptom.

A number of studies of non-primate mammals have demonstrated
an inverse relationship between an animal's control over hazardous
environments and fear. Mowrer and Viek in 1948 reported that
rats exposed to inescapable shock later showed deficits in escape-
avoidance learning. Mowrer's two-stage learning theory proposed
that psychopathology is a function of both classical conditioning
(based on associative relationships) and instrumental learning whereby individuals will avoid conditioned cues evoking anxiety (Keane
et al. 1985). A rat hearing a bell ringing (the conditioned stimulus)
shortly before receiving an electric shock (the unconditioned stimulus) comes to fear the sound of the bell (the conditioned response). If
the rat subsequently learns that a particular corner of its cage is
immune from electric shocks when the bell rings, it learns to use this
corner as a haven.

Eysenck and Rachman (1965) proposed an avoidance-learning
model of phobic conditioning in humans in which classically conditioned fear results in avoidance responses, which are then reinforced

by a reduction in fear. This remains a cornerstone of clinical practice, including my own, but its shortcomings are frequently ignored.

Rats reared in contingent environments (i.e. those in which they had a degree of control) were found to be less emotional following experimental treatment (Joffe et al. 1973). However, importantly the study could not answer the question of whether control decreased emotionality, or whether lack of control increased it. In another study rats chose signalled shock in inescapable/unavoidable shock situations versus unsignalled similarly aversive stimuli. This was probably because they could relax while there was no danger signal, a finding consistent with a safety signal hypothesis. The safety signal hypothesis simply refers to experimental animals being given notice that they can relax for a while before their next shocks. Rats also preferred information on the nature of the shock, i.e. what to expect. Greater fear is induced when the fear stimulus occurs in a context previously signalling safety. In other words if the time out ceases to be safe, the situation is perceived as more anxiety provoking. However, several reports seemed to contradict the safety signal hypothesis (Fanselow 1980). Nevertheless, it is now well recognized that PTSD in humans is more likely when safety beliefs are shattered, for example in children abused by their fathers (Foa et al. 1992).

A more realistic conditioning model for human psychopathology, especially PTSD, may require a number of conditioned stimuli. This more complex conditioning scenario may involve 'higher order conditioning'. This involves pairing an initial conditioned stimulus (e.g. a bell) with a second conditioned stimulus (e.g. a buzzer), which becomes a (higher order) conditioned stimulus in its own right. Stimulus generalization suggests that the closer the new stimulus is to the first, the stronger its response will be. Higher order conditioning and stimulus generalization could account for the wide range of stimuli that evoke traumatic memories in people with PTSD (Keane et al. 1985).

Repeatedly defeated mice have been found to experience decreased pain perception to heat inflicted on their tails (Miczec et al. 1982). Results suggested endogenous opioid mediated analgesia activated the stress of such defeat. Opioid-like analgesia subsequently has been found to be a feature of PTSD in humans (Pitman et al. 1990).

Some studies found reduced aggression associated with fear stimuli, inconsistent with the increased aggression of PTSD, emphasizing the need for caution in drawing conclusions from studies designed for exploring normal anxiety responses. For example, Scott and

Marston (1953) found that after four to six days of serial defeats, most selectively bred fighting mice could not be trained to fight within a two-week period: defeats produced persistent inhibition of fighting. However, using a different experimental design, mice receiving shocks have been found to become aggressive. Pynoos and colleagues (1996) described: 'Between the third and sixth week, excessive fighting erupted that resulted in the death or maiming of all animals in a cage.' Regrettably, it is unclear how many occupied the cage and little other information was provided, as aggression was not the focus of the study.

Learned helplessness

Overmier and Seligman (1967) and Seligman and Maier (1967) followed on from Mowrer and Viek's (1948) early work and found that exposure of dogs to inescapable shocks under various conditions interfered with subsequent instrumental escape-avoidance responding in new situations. Dogs exposed to shocks when released from their harnesses behaved passively, failing to learn escape responses. Subsequently Seligman (1975) suggested the influential phenomenon he called 'learned helplessness' applied to a variety of species. Controllability is central to the learned helplessness paradigm. A number of neurochemical changes associated with learned helplessness were described (Anisman 1978). Inescapable shock may produce learned helplessness via learned decreases in general activity, from neurochemical depletion or both (Jackson et al. 1980).

The 1970s was an era when conditioning researchers believed that behaviour could be scientifically observed and measured but thoughts could not. Hence, they preferred to disregard the existence of thoughts as being too nebulous to be worth bothering about. Yet, behaviourists later rediscovered thoughts inventing a new growth industry called cognitive behaviour therapy, which is the dominant psychological paradigm of the present time. However, Wortman and Brehm (1975) integrated helplessness and reactance theories suggesting that when individuals initially lose control, they become motivated to regain control, but with extended exposure they give up. This cognitive as opposed to behavioural model challenged the learned helplessness concept.

Repeated defeat of rats by other rats has been found to produce similar responses to learned helplessness from electric shocks. Dominant colony male rats given inescapable shocks showed increased defensive responses, but virtually no customary aggression when later tested with naive conspecific (same species) intruders (Williams and Lierle 1988). Williams and Lierle (1988) described a stress-coping-fear-defence theory, which suggests that inescapable shocks produce greater fear to contextual stimuli than escapable shocks. Rats exposed to repeated defeat showed defensive and/or submissive responses, receiving increased numbers of bites when acting as intruders.

These findings of submissiveness at first appear to contradict any evolutionary suggestion of adaptiveness. However, this illusion is a product of abnormal research environments. In the wild a submissive animal does not usually invade a dominant's territory. These findings are consistent with the more recent ethological observations of 'blocked escape' (Gilbert 1992). An animal whose escape is blocked (e.g. by not being able to leave the security of its group because of predation risk) remains in a stressful situation. If that animal is a subordinate who has repeatedly been defeated, it would do well to behave in a respectful and submissive manner in the presence of a dominant. However, I am running ahead of myself.

Controllability and predictability

The concepts of controllability and predictability are fundamental to understanding PTSD (Foa et al. 1992). Escape or blocked escape are obviously related to controllability. Controllability is so intimately linked with the concept of predictability that it is a mistake to examine either in isolation. An organism that has control over an event has some degree of predictability over when it will end (Wortman and Brehm 1975). Conversely while some predictable events may not be directly controllable, signals preceding aversive events may allow organisms to prepare for the events. The hum of the dentist's drill may not be avoidable but it permits you to hang on tight. Signals also provide information on when shocks will not occur. You can relax when the drill noise stops.

Mineka and Hendersen (1985) reviewed studies of uncontrollable versus controllable shock in animals and humans. Uncontrollable shocks have resulted in behavioural changes in animals such as lower aggression and competition, and in humans have resulted in impaired problem solving and increased passivity. Animals have demonstrated conditioning of fear to neutral stimuli paired with shock, while humans report mood changes such as anxiety.

In uncontrollably shocked animals, physiological changes have included increased stress-induced ulceration, opiate-mediated analgesia, suppression of lymphocyte proliferation, susceptibility to certain cancers, the production of antibodies (Laudenslager et al. 1988) and alterations in cortisol and neurotransmitter levels. Zoo animals have been found to be healthier when they have to work for food and other reinforcers, even when a net loss of reinforcement results.

The effects of perceived control appear similar to those with actual control. Generally, mastery has been less studied but the evidence suggests findings opposite to those of learned helplessness. Experience with control leads to mastery, with animals persevering in trying to control uncontrollable shocks. The same principle applies in children, with helplessness-orientated children tending to forget their successes. Hence, controllability research needs to be considered at a number of levels including behavioural, physiological and cognitive (Mineka and Hendersen 1985).

Mineka et al. (1986) compared operant (learning by way of rewards and punishments) versus non-operant conditioning in rhesus monkeys. These monkeys had been provided with contingent or non-contingent rewards such as access to food, water and treats from their second month of life. Operant subjects later showed less fear and more exploratory behaviour. Others have observed that loss of control tends to be more stressful than lack of control (Foa et al. 1992). Having some control over the termination of the traumatic experience greatly reduces conditioning of fear (Mineka and Zinbarg 1991). Further prior control/mastery experiences in rhesus monkeys have been associated with less fear (Mineka et al. 1986).

Flaws of overly simplistic conditioning theories

Learning even at emotional and behavioural levels need not be direct – it may involve observation. Monkeys that have observed non-fearful monkeys behave non-fearfully in response to a variety of snake stimuli, later were found to experience reduced fear conditioning via subsequent observation of monkeys behaving fearfully with snakes (Mineka and Cook 1986).

In primates facial expression has a major role in communication, especially in relation to fear. Social fears conditioned in primates by angry faces directed at observer primates were found to be much more resistant to extinction than other emotion facial conditioning

(Ohman 1986). Angry facial expression serves an important signalling function that symbolizes violence, usually without the need to employ it, thereby saving all concerned from injuries that could threaten survival. Even trivial injuries occasionally become infected, with life-threatening consequences.

Early conditioning studies naively assumed that life presents us with a blank slate onto which experience is conditioned. However, observer rhesus monkeys can be easily conditioned to acquire a fear of snakes but not of flowers (Cook and Mineka 1987). While much predator defence in birds is innate, observational learning has been similarly demonstrated in laboratory experimentation (Curio 1988). Hence, the simple classical conditioning model needs modification to cater for the fact that certain associations are innately more easily conditioned than others and observational learning, which may be influenced not only by behaviour but also by signals associated with facial expression.

Other major flaws exist with overly simplistic conditioning models of phobic avoidance. Experiential variables have tended to assume that organisms of the same species are all the same, neglecting the influences of life experiences and genetic variation (Mineka and Zinbarg 1991). Safe previous experiences may dramatically retard fear conditioning. Behavioural inhibition is the temperamental construct most relevant to anxiety. It also displays significant genetic variation.

Another problem is that phobias commonly occur in people with no history of traumatic conditioning history (Mineka and Cook 1993). Further, phobias are remarkably resistant to extinction, considerably more so than laboratory-conditioned fears.

Mineka and Zinbarg (1991) suggested that controllability research may be considered as providing 'mini models', which do not explain the full phobic syndrome but may provide insights into parts of it. This seems especially relevant when extrapolating such findings to PTSD.

A further problem with traditional conditioning models has been their failure to consider the dynamic context. Mineka and Zinbarg (1995) have referred to this deficiency as the 'Stress-in-Total-Isolation Anxiety Model' and contrasted it with a 'Stress-in-Dynamic-Context Anxiety Model'. Context includes temperament, past experiences, current context and future context.

Preparedness

With little doubt the greatest flaw posed by overly simplistic conditioning notions was that associated with what Seligman (1971) called 'preparedness' – genetically facilitated learning. Garcia et al. (1968) performed an interesting early study. Four groups of rodents were tested regarding four variables associated with food pellets – size and flavour of pellet, paired with malaise induced by X-rays or pain due to electric shock. When electric shock was paired with the size of the pellet eaten, rats quickly learnt to avoid the size associated with shock. However, even though rats were shocked immediately after beginning to eat the wrong flavoured food, they did not learn to associate the flavour with electric shocks. By contrast, when food was paired with X-ray treatment – which induced illness an hour later – rats quickly learnt to avoid the flavoured food associated with illness. However, they did not learn to associate size of pellet eaten with illness. Flavour was easily associated with sickness, but the size of pellet was not. Furthermore, when sickness was induced with X-rays as long as twelve hours after feeding, the rats were still successfully aversively conditioned to the flavour of food items. Natural selection favours efficient means of learning what 'foods' are safe to eat. Taste but not pellet size relates to the chemical composition of food. Animals may learn such associations despite long delays between the stimuli and punishment.

Bolles (1970) was rightly critical of early research for being out of touch with what was known about animal defence in nature. He suggested that animals have species-specific defence reactions, e.g. specific approaches to fleeing, freezing and fighting. If an avoidance response is rapidly learnt then it must be a species-specific defence reaction. Innate potential facilitates rapid learning. Prey animals cannot afford to have a learning system that requires the experience of tangible and repeated pain from predators. A mechanism for learning that does not require multiple exposures is of great survival value (Silove 1998). Many experimental studies of avoidance learning may be more valid to slowly acquired responses. As these do not have the resistance to extinction associated with phobias and PTSD, this is a major limitation for conditioning research.

Seligman's (1971) theory of preparedness suggests that primates and humans have phylogenetically based predispositions to rapidly acquire fears relevant to our ancestral history – favouring those who rapidly acquired them. The preparedness phenomenon was initially viewed by many as more an obstacle to research than a fascinating research issue in its own right.

Not everyone ignored the challenge of preparedness research. Cook and Mineka (1989) noted that fears and phobias of snakes, spiders and heights are common, but such fears of hammers, electrical outlets or guns are not, even though the latter are associated with greater danger. However, preparedness still may require learning. Laboratory-reared monkeys were not initially afraid of snakes but rapidly became so after observing wild-reared monkeys, which were afraid of snakes. To test the possibility that the fear reaction itself might account for the strength of the learnt reaction, Cook and Mineka asked the question 'Would comparable conditioning occur if models were seen reacting fearfully to fear-irrelevant stimuli?' First, they checked that observers would acquire fear when viewing models responding fearfully to fear-relevant stimuli via viewing video footage – they did. Then, by cutting and splicing tapes, they found that viewers acquired fears only when viewing fear reactions of models responding to fear-relevant stimuli (e.g. snakes). There was little response to observed fear reactions paired with irrelevant stimuli such as flowers. Further, laboratory-reared viewer monkeys had no prior experience with snakes or flowers; hence the acquired fears must be phylogenetic rather than ontogenetic in origin.

Evolutionarily relevant fears are conditioned far more quickly and extinguish far more slowly than fear-irrelevant stimuli (Ohman 1986). Fawns are not born with fears of wolves, but lifelong panic may be conditioned by only once seeing their mothers flee from wolves (Marks and Nesse 1997). Ohman and Soares (1994) found that subliminal fear-relevant (but not irrelevant) conditioned stimuli could generate conditioned responses. They also suggested that phobics might be unable to control fear because its origin is in cognitive structures controlled by non-conscious mechanisms. This is of immense relevance to the irrationality of PTSD.

Arne Ohman and Susan Mineka (and their colleagues) have conducted many years of research in this area and comprehensively reviewed the literature relating to humans and monkeys. The result has been their developing 'an evolved module of fear learning' (Ohman and Mineka 2001). This has four characteristics:

(a) The fear module is preferentially activated in aversive contexts by stimuli that are fear relevant in an evolutionary perspective. (b) Its activation to such stimuli is automatic. (c) It is relatively impenetrable to cognitive control. (d) It originates in a dedicated neural circuitry, centred on the amygdala.

Point (a) relates to selectively sensitive learning responses to stimuli that have been correlated with threatening encounters in the evolutionary past. Virtually all animals contend with predators and defence against them must be a priority.

Automaticity is far more rapid than cognitive processing could allow for. Human cognitive superiority would be a liability in threatening situations where survival responses are measured in fractions of or a few seconds. More basic preconscious brain processing inherited from our less cognitively inclined ancestry is quicker (Ohman and Mineka 2001).

A third characteristic of the module is its relative 'encapsulation' from, or inpenetrability to, other brain influences; once initiated, severe fear tends to run its course with modest potential for modification by cognitive influences (Ohman and Mineka 2001). The dominant influence of the amygdala is covered in the following subsection.

Ohman and Mineka's (2001) review is far more comprehensive than my limited space can do justice to. Nevertheless, some challenges to their theory of selective *associative* learning is required. Another possibility is the selective *sensitization* hypothesis, in which fear-relevant stimuli are genetically encoded directly to elicit fear, but a state of anxiety or arousal is required for manifestations of fear to emerge. A newborn's first breaths result from anoxia and constitution as opposed to associative learning. They concede that selective sensitization may occur, but only selective associative learning is long lasting as found in phobias. The latter is consistent with observations that laboratory-reared monkeys need to learn snake fear for this instinct to become active.

Preparedness is so important that I will risk labouring the point with another illustration, this time from the natural world of animal learning of non-traumatic survival responses. Trivers (1985) has commented:

> Far from having a single general ability to learn, animals have a variety of more or less specific learning abilities, each tailored to natural selection to a particular task. . . . Consider the way male birds sing. . . . In order to develop his species-typical song, a male bird must hear other birds singing. He usually has the

innate ability to recognize his own species' song and memorizes it in preference to others. In some species the sensitive period for such learning is over long before the male actually begins to sing, so the bird does not learn to sing through simple imitation . . . once the bird starts to sing, he listens to what he sings and tries to match it to the song he has earlier memorized. . . . The accuracy of the mimicry also varies – from species in which copying is very extensive to ones in which only elements are copied.

On that tuneful note we will move on.

Observations from combat and torture

When considering these fear-conditioning findings with respect to human traumatization, it is of interest to note that strains on guerrilla forces, such as in the Vietnam War, stem in part from inability to distinguish non-combatants and enemy – i.e. unpredictability (Laufer et al. 1985). Human torturers attempt to maximize unpredictability and uncontrollability and block mastery. Further, torturers use isolation as it reduces the reassurance associated with safety signals. Nakedness may be used to promote a sense of helplessness. Another deliberately damaging tactic is being kept waiting for a torture session and/or being given a false time of the next torture experience (lack of predictability) (Basoglu and Mineka 1992). Conversely captives staging hunger strikes experience a sense of control. Resisting torture by not crying out, for example, or by feeding the torturers false information may further enhance a victim's sense of control. Controllability and predictability remain very relevant to PTSD despite all the problems with oversimplistic interpretations of conditioning observations.

Controllability and PTSD

Let us now turn to the much less extensive research on controllability that is specific to PTSD. Uncontrollable and/or unpredictable shocks have been found to have remarkably consistent effects across the then four DSM-III-R symptom categories of arousal, re-experiencing, numbing and avoidance (numbing now being in the avoidance group of DSM-IV) (Foa et al. 1992).

   PTSD symptoms of victims of criminal assault have been found to be more severe if the trauma was perceived as 'generally' uncontrollable (Kushner et al. 1992). Although it is established that the severity of a trauma is related to the risk of developing PTSD symptoms, perceived controllability was found to be largely independent of assault characteristics with respect to PTSD severity. Only the level of force (not severity of injuries, etc.) correlated with perceived control. Psychopathology appears more severe when perceived lack of control is generalized beyond the attack. This concurs with the observation that problems emerge when basic assumptions about the fairness and safety of the world in general are violated (Janoff-Bulman and Frieze 1983).

Some of the symptoms of PTSD may be mutually or self-reinforcing. Anger is incompatible with anxiety and so angry expressions may diminish anxiety, reinforcing anger as a coping behaviour. Avoidance of talking about traumas limits the potential exposure during which extinction might occur (Keane et al. 1985). On the other hand, avoiding talking about traumatic experiences with those unlikely to be able to understand and respond appropriately may reduce secondary traumatization. Rape victims may experience secondary traumatization if sharing their experience is met with derision.

Summary

All mammals can be conditioned to new fear stimuli with relatively similar results. However, evolutionarily relevant fear stimuli produce much more rapid and enduring conditioning results than irrelevant stimuli. This phenomenon is known as preparedness and involves the innate facilitation of learning important for defence and other selection pressures. It reflects our ancestral history. The original classical and operant conditioning models failed to adequately recognize the importance of preparedness. Phobic behaviours including PTSD differ from conditioned fears in several important respects: when phobias are acquired through traumatic conditioning they often need only one trial; phobias are much more resistant to extinction; traumatic conditioned phobias are often associated with a long delay between the conditioned stimulus and the unconditioned stimulus; phobias tend to relate to evolutionarily selected objects, and phobias are more irrational and resistant to cognitive change. Nevertheless, partial control or prior mastery of the problem decreases fear conditioning. The controllability and predictability of aversive stimuli such as fear are important factors offsetting psychopathology. The absence of controllability and predictability is central to the concepts of learned helplessness, blocked escape – and PTSD.

MYOPIA AND TWENTY-FIRST CENTURY NEUROSCIENCE

> Science is facts; just as houses are made of stones, so is science made of facts; but a pile of stones is not a house and a collection of facts is not necessarily science.
>
> Henri Poincaré, 1854–1912

Proximate versus distal perspectives

Recent advances in biological treatments of mental symptoms have led many to the premature conclusion that neurophysiological 'defects' underlie most mental disorders. This notion neglects the possible adaptive function of the associated behaviours (Nesse 1997). Cough, diarrhoea and vomiting are symptoms of illness, yet they evolved to eliminate noxious substances. While under some conditions suppression of these symptoms may be beneficial, under others it may prolong the illnesses. Numerous neurophysiological abnormalities have been found in PTSD. From the proximal perspective of the impaired individual, these may be considered abnormalities. However, from the more distal evolutionary perspective, it is likely that at least some changes might be considered adaptive – mostly in our ancestral past. Occasionally, even nowadays they might be adaptive, for example a mountaineer who 'lost his nerve' following a climb in which friends died. Also in the present time, if PTSD exists on a continuum with normality, subclinical symptoms could well be advantageous, such as a lucky escape from a motor vehicle accident with ongoing unease deterring the individual from driving too fast.

I will continue next with the neuroscientific work of Paul MacLean and Jaak Panksepp, who have not received the recognition from psychiatry that is warranted. Their works serve the key function of bridging the proximal and distal orientations.

The triune brain

In 1949 Paul MacLean published his concept of 'the triune brain' – a three-level brain concept (Figure 3.1). He suggested that the human forebrain evolved and expanded to its great size, while retaining features of three basic evolutionary formations, reflecting ancestral relationships to reptiles (which predated mammals by 100 million years), early mammals and recent mammals. His conceptualization divided the development of the human brain according to this evolutionary timeframe and according to fundamental neuroanatomy, with newer structures evolving around older inner structures.

MacLean (1949) conceptualized the innermost and oldest parts of human brains as 'reptilian', reflecting their early development. Reptilian functions are mostly behavioural and reflexive. The middle

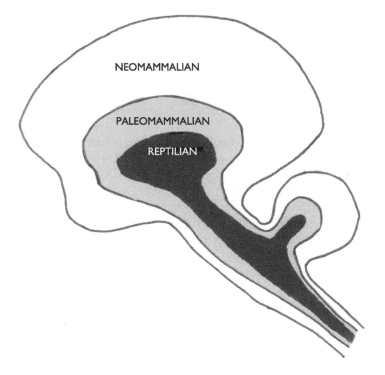

Figure 3.1 MacLean's triune brain
Source: *The Triune Brain in Evolution: role in paleocerebral functions* (Figure 2.1) by MacLean (1990). Reprinted with kind permission of Springer Science and Business Media.

'paleomammalian' (older mammalian) layers are largely emotions orientated. The most recent outer 'neomammalian' (newer mammalian) layers are responsible for cognition. Intercommunication between the areas may occur while operating somewhat independently. In response to an unexpected danger a person may reflexively freeze, become afraid and then consider the threat logically.

The reptilian brain involves the basal ganglia and extrapyramidal motor system responsible for behavioural responses to emotional systems including fear, anger, sexuality and other primitive but essential survival functions (MacLean 1949). Anatomically the reptilian core is relatively uniform (proportionally) in size in all mammals (Panksepp 1998). Emotional systems energize and guide organisms in their interactions with their environments. The primitive emotions of reptiles provided the context-dependent drive, but their lack of self-awareness would greatly limit any subjective emotional experience, which we refer to as 'feelings'.

The old mammalian brain saw the development of the limbic system, although it is not a discrete anatomical entity. This paleomammalian development involved major advances in emotional systems serving adaptive behaviours. These emotions bring greater awareness of feelings and motivation for interacting with environmental events (Panksepp 1998).

The neocortex is small in rodents, which emerged early in mammalian evolution, and massive in the more recent cetaceans (whales) and the great apes, especially humans. While the limbic system is our feeling brain, the neocortex is our thinking brain. It receives sensory stimuli, analyses them and interacts with the external world, solving problems through conscious rational experience. This is a tardy process involving delaying or suppressing action while imagining it. It brings the benefit of complex considerations in decision-making, but cannot exist without the basic but more rapid subcortical and more determined limbic defences. While the neocortex can be moved by and rationally influence emotions, it cannot generate them without the ancient subcortical functions (Panksepp 1998).

Phobias are experienced as a dissociation between fear and cognition, overwhelming fear that is accepted as irrational, demonstrating the relative separation of primitive defence-related emotions from thoughts (Ohman and Mineka 2001). This separation can be further illustrated by backward-masking techniques. A target stimulus is very briefly presented to subjects, then followed by a second masking stimulus for somewhat longer. Subjects are able to guess the presentations of subliminal fear versus neutral stimuli without being able to recall them (Ohman and Mineka 2001). Furthermore, they can be conditioned to subliminal fear stimuli, especially biologically relevant ones, despite their lack of awareness.

Self-awareness is one of the recent neocortical developments. It allows animals to predict the social responses of their conspecifics. Self-awareness positively exploded with the advent of *Homo sapiens* and the most recent model, *Homo sapiens sapiens*. Neocortical functions include self-preservation and more complex social bonding (MacLean 1990; Schelde and Hertz 1994). The latter gave rise to cooperative behaviour, which took defence in the more recent mammals to a new group level.

Twenty-first century?

Following on from Paul MacLean, Jaak Panksepp (1998, 2000) has called for a coming together of neurology and psychology via an evolution-based approach to brain studies. He has emphasized humans sharing with mammals many basic evolved psychoneural processes, which energize and guide organisms in their interactions with the world. He suggests the dichotomy between thinking and feeling is a fundamental distinction, not just a poetic metaphor.

A superficial misconception of the limbic system is to view it as an emotions centre. There is no emotions centre; instead there is circuitry. Panksepp (1998, 2000) has proposed a preliminary taxonomy of distinct emotional modular systems, supported by neuroscientific findings. First, reflexive affects are sited principally low in the brainstem – for example the startle reflex, gustatory disgust, pain, hunger and so on. Second, there are what he calls 'grade-A emotions' that are situated in the intermediate areas of the brain. These are conceptualized as sensorimotor emotional command circuits, the consequences of which may outlast the triggering conditions – for example fear, anger, sadness, joy, affection and interest. Third, there are the higher sentiments associated with the recent expansion of the forebrain, including shame, guilt, contempt, envy, humour, empathy, sympathy and certain forms of jealousy. In PTSD deep subcortical networks become sensitized and operate independently of higher cortical faculties. Behavioural and emotional responses may be activated in situations that do not make neocortical sense. One of the most universal symptoms of PTSD is feeling unsafe in public. Cues from the numbers of people around activate primitive withdrawal behaviours and the emotion fear – that cognitively appear absurd.

Panksepp has proposed and named the following grade-A emotions with their names in capitals and relevant functions in lower case: SEEKING/expectancy, RAGE/anger, FEAR/anxiety, LUST/sexuality, CARE/nurturance, PANIC/separation and PLAY/joy. RAGE and FEAR systems so central to PTSD are so closely related that some researchers suggest they are one – a defence module. However, Panksepp (1998, 2000) suggests they are separate. RAGE areas include the medial amygdala to the bed nucleus of the stria terminalis, and medial and perifornical hypothalamus to dorsal periaqueductal grey matter. FEAR key areas include the central and lower amygdala to medial hypothalamus and dorsal periaqueductal grey matter.

Three distinct aggressive circuits in the mammalian brain exist – predatory, intermale/interconspecific (relating to dominance struggles) and RAGE (Panksepp 1998). When humans go hunting they may feel aggressive but they are not consumed by anger. In the run-up to a boxing bout, anger may benefit from neocortical cultivation. With true rage aggression is driven by a tornado, which needs no help from the neocortex. Affective rage and defensive aggression may involve piloerection but predatory aggression does not, illustrating neurophysiological differences.

All mammalian behaviour is a mix of innate and learned components, approximately equally proportioned in humans (Panksepp 1998, 2000). Laboratory-reared rats exhibit fear responses to the smell of cats and other predators even though they have never encountered them before. Genetic and learned aspects of behaviour may be separate but are intimately related. For example, young birds do not so much learn *to fly* (this is innate) but they do learn *where to* fly. Practically all brain systems change with use and disuse.

The core symptoms of PTSD relate more directly to the two more primitive brain areas. The neocortex is mostly a witness to the confusing responses arising from reptilian and paleomammalian brain levels. Decorticate animals (whose higher centres have been rendered surgically functionless for experiments) can still respond emotionally, but they have decreased ability to regulate their emotions. Decorticate animals still exhibit escape and fear behaviours. Higher brain functions are desirable but their absence does not preclude such survival responses (Panksepp 1998). The interconnectedness of the three brain levels promotes mixing of lower behaviours and emotions with cognitive processes. A car backfiring may instantaneously alarm an ordinary individual, whose emotions will quickly subside with higher cortical appraisal. Those with PTSD not only are more easily alarmed, but also despite neocortical logic remain disturbed and confused by ongoing activity from intermediate brain regions.

Facial emotions

> When a woman is talking to you, listen to what she says with her eyes.
>
> Victor Hugo, 1802–1885

A remarkably large area of the human brain is allocated to the interpretation of facial expressions (Panksepp 1998). This is because conspecific communication accounts for a large proportion of brain activity and so much is communicated by facial responses (Gardner and Wilson 2004). Our ability to verbally describe facial communicative expressions is far outweighed by our ability to be influenced by them. Our paleocortex greatly outperforms our neocortex in this respect. This is a vivid illustration of the relative separation of limbic and neocortical analysis of emotional and facial communication. It also illustrates the importance of non-verbal communication and non-cognitive interpretation of the environment with respect to essential evolutionary tasks.

Facial expressions have served an important signalling function between conspecifics, long predating the emergence of language controlled by the neocortex (Panksepp 1998). Facial expression is a means of communication in many mammals but particularly complex in humans despite our availability of language. The evolution of human social complexity and non-verbal communication may have become sufficiently replete that language developed.

Much of emotional experience occurs outside of our awareness. The right amygdala is important for facial threat detection as demonstrated by neural responses elicited in the right (but not left) amygdala to masked presentations of a conditioned angry face (Morris et al. 1998). Bearing this in mind consider the following experimental findings. Esteves and Ohman (1993) used fleeting (33 millisecond) presentations of fearful and happy facial expressions followed immediately with longer (167 millisecond) presentations of neutral faces. Most subjects 'saw' the longer presentations of neutral faces but not the briefer presentations of fearful or happy faces. Nevertheless, amygdala functional magnetic resonance imaging signal activity was greater with the 'unseen' fearful faces, despite subjects reporting no effects on their emotional arousal. This suggests that the amygdala may monitor the environment for positive and negative stimuli and that reported emotions and amygdala activation should not be equated (Davis and Whalen 2001).

The amygdala may increase vigilance by lowering neuronal thresholds in sensory systems. Fearful faces are more ambiguous than angry faces as while an angry face signals threat, a fearful face signals that a threat is nearby to be found. Hypervigilance is a key feature of PTSD. From their neuroscientific perspective, Davis and Whalen (2001) proposed: 'Pathological anxiety may not be a disorder of fear, but a disorder of vigilance.'

Essential neuroanatomy of PTSD

The relevance of the following section on neuroanatomy is not so much in drawing a map of the brain, but in demonstrating that brain functioning is not simply input, followed by thinking – including unconscious and conscious – and then choice of response. The brain is far more mysterious and complicated. Neuroanatomy I have found is a bit like reading a Russian novel. Fascinating, but frustrating. If only I could reliably remember all those unfamiliar names. For readers unfamiliar with brain anatomy and for those feeling a bit rusty, I start this section with a simple overview of the essential brain structures relevant to PTSD and their functions. If you get lost, please return to the following summary paragraph to reorientate yourself.

The sensory organs provide sensory input to the thalamus. The thalamus acts as an incoming sensory relay station sending on selected integrated sensory information to the prefrontal cortex, which is a part of the brain's higher centres for thoughts. The thalamus diverts sensory information of emotional significance to the amygdala, which in simple terms has been thought of as a fear centre, although I will revise this later. The amygdala interprets the emotional significance of this incoming information. It registers emotional memories and may recall them without conscious awareness of their significance. The amygdala also relays emotionally significant messages to the hippocampus. The hippocampus has a major role in the learning of emotionally significant and spatial and temporal issues and the conscious recall of them. It's not much use to remember that you previously spotted a predator, unless you have details such as when and where. Recall of contextual details promotes survival. The hippocampus relays such learnt material on to the prefrontal cortex where such memory is stored. The prefrontal cortex acting as a reservoir of relevant stored knowledge can provide a relatively slow supply of knowledge back to the amygdala directly or via the hippocampus, which may modify amygdala activity (van der Kolk 1996b). For example, in fear situations it may relay messages such as 'Yes, it is a snake, but it is not a poisonous one.' The amygdala also relays messages to the hypothalamus and to the basal forebrain for motor activity. This slower indirect route of fear registration activates a complex endocrine response for purposes of flight or fight.

The thalamus is the key sensory input relay station. It relays sensory information to the basal ganglia where it effects movement, to the limbic system where it generates memories and emotions and to the cerebral cortex where it produces thoughts (van der Kolk 1996c). If such input is identified as relevant to survival, the thalamus can serve as a quicker but cruder unconscious sensory centre than the cortex. It relays such information to the amygdala for a rapid response. Hence there are two routes for emotional learning – cortical (conscious but slow) and subcortical (unconscious but fast). We would all have died long ago if we relied on our slow-witted conscious processes for day-to-day hazard avoidance. Subcortical memory simply needs to be able to store primitive cues and detect them. Later, coordination of this basic information with the cortex permits verification (LeDoux 2002).

The limbic system reflects the paleomammalian phase of MacLean's model of brain evolution and development. Virtually all researchers and clinicians agree on the limbic system's importance, yet we remain uncertain about what its structural boundaries should be. The amygdala may be the most important limbic structure, yet Davis and Whalen (2001) state that 'including the basolateral nucleus with certain surrounding nuclei [of the amygdala] such as the central, medial and cortical nuclei, into a single entity does not make anatomical sense.' It gets worse; we can suggest some of the limbic system's functions, but by no means all of them. The demonstrable importance of the amygdala in fear conditioning, is probably the reason for the limbic system's ongoing use (LeDoux and Phelps 2000). However, even this I will later suggest may need to be re-evaluated. Nevertheless, it seems clear that the amygdala, especially the basolateral amygdala, is essential for assigning feelings to sensory input, prior to their elaboration by the neocortex (van der Kolk 1996c).

The amygdala is a major interface for sensory and cognitive input regarding stressors and for the emerging behavioural responses. The timeframe for this response is several milliseconds. It involves stimulation of the solitary tract for parasympathetic responses, projections to the lateral hypothalamus and then rostral ventral medulla for sympathetic responses (flight or fight), projections from the central amygdala to the bed nucleus of the stria terminalis to initiate the hypothalamo-pituitary adrenal (HPA) axis response, and other processes (Yehuda 1999). The central nucleus of the amygdala is involved in the startle reflex (Krystal et al. 1989). Significantly, the amygdala has denser efferent than afferent connections with the cortex, suggesting that fear affects cognition more than the reverse (LeDoux 1996). The fear responses of our ancestry are called upon, in preference to modern logic.

Outputs to the hippocampus influence the development of conscious memories of emotional events as well as modulating spatial learning. Connections with cortical areas may be involved in the representation of positive or negative rewards in memory to guide choice behaviour (Davis and Whalen 2001). Broadly speaking, while the amygdala serves fear learning, the hippocampus serves cognitive learning (Ohman and Mineka 2001).

The basolateral amygdala connections to the central nucleus of the amygdala along with the latter's outgoing projections represent a central fear system (Davis and Whalen 2001). In particular these connections mediate autonomic and somatic signs of fear and attention to significant stimuli. The lateral extended amygdala projections to the central grey matter appear to be a critical part of a general defence system. They have been implicated in freezing and stress-induced analgesia. Stimulation of the central nucleus of the amygdala produces a cessation of ongoing behaviour, a component of the freezing response.

LeDoux et al. (1989) have demonstrated that the classical conditioning of fear reactions to acoustic stimuli is mediated by projections from auditory processing areas of the thalamus, bypassing the auditory cortex to the amygdala – constituting a subcortical mechanism of emotional learning – i.e. sounds are registered and responded to by the brain, without conscious awareness. This occurs despite the thalamus being the major sensory relay station to the cortex. If acoustic stimuli are of sufficient importance, e.g. loud or unusual, the rapid direct route to the amygdala may take priority over the slower conscious cortical route.

LeDoux et al. (1989) also found that visual conditioning in animals does not depend on the integrity of the visual cortex. Animals could be cortically blind but still respond to visual stimuli. Further, emotional memories established in the absence of a visual cortex were remarkably persistent, resisting extinction. The visual cortex may be important for promoting extinction by relaying information to the frontal cortex, hippocampus and other areas. This would include information that the aforementioned snake is not a poisonous one. Thalamo-amygdala projections may be involved in visual as well as auditory fear conditioning.

The amygdala has different regions for different functions. The lateral nucleus of the amygdala is the sensory interface in fear conditioning. It receives inputs from the auditory thalamus. The central nucleus functions as an interface for responses. Lesions of the central nucleus block fear-potentiated startle, while electrical stimulation of the central nucleus increases acoustic startle (Bremner et al. 1999). However, the lateral nucleus can influence the central nucleus via the basolateral nucleus, accessory basal or basomedial nucleus (LeDoux 2002). In rats the central nucleus of amygdala has been shown to control fear-related blood pressure changes, freezing and startle reactions. The basolateral amygdala is involved in negative and positive mood as well as spatial and motor learning (Davis and Whalen 2001).

The hippocampus has a key role in processing fear and anxiety-related information about the environment. It selects spatial and temporal dimensions of experience for storage in memory (van der Kolk 1996b; Bremner et al. 1999). The hippocampus also assesses new information as to whether it involves reward, punishment, novelty or non-reward. Significant information is passed on to the prefrontal cortex for memory storage. The amygdala plays a major role in modulating the storage and strength of memories based on their emotional and thus survival relevance (LeDoux 2002). Traumatic memories may emerge as affect states, somatic sensations, or visual images that are timeless and unmodified by further experience (van der Kolk 1994). In animals hippocampal lesions after fear conditioning prevent the expression of responses to surroundings (LeDoux 2002). Upsets in infants and toddlers may be felt as exemplified by tears of distress, but not later recalled because the hippocampus is slow to mature for conscious memories (LeDoux 2002).

The process by which the hippocampus selects and relays memories to the cortex for long-term storage is lengthy. The hippocampus may repeatedly relay such memories to the cortex over about two years, with these relays serving the function of consolidating the memory traces in the cortex that otherwise might be prone to being erased (Carter 1998). Experiments with rats suggest that during slow wave sleep, synaptic modification within the hippocampus is suppressed and the neuronal states encoded within the hippocampus are replayed as part of a consolidation process by which hippocampal information is gradually transferred to the neocortex (Wilson and McNaughton 1994).

Contextual fear association learning not only involves but also may alter the hippocampus. Children with PTSD who have suffered severe childhood physical and sexual abuse have been found to show a 12 per cent decrease in left hippocampal volume (Bremner et al. 1999). Hippocampal atrophy has been found in combat veterans with PTSD with a correlation between combat exposure and hippocampal volume. Glucocorticoid toxicity may result in atrophy of parts of the hippocampus (Yehuda 1999). Glucocorticoids control genes for cognitive integration and memory and circadian rhythms. Hippocampal atrophy may involve toxic effects of cortisol at the time of trauma or increase the number or sensitivity of glucocorticoid receptors (Graham et al. 1999; Yehuda 1999; McEwen 2000; De Bellis 2001).

An alternative explanation is that smaller hippocampal volume (perhaps due to earlier stressors) might predispose to PTSD (Graham et al. 1999). Support for this suggestion has recently emerged. A magnetic resonance imaging (MRI) study of forty monozygotic (identical) twin pairs, in which one of each pair was a Vietnam veteran, found that men without combat exposure demonstrated similarly reduced hippocampal volumes to those of their combat-exposed PTSD-suffering twins. Both such twins had smaller hippocampal volumes than combat-exposed non-PTSD sufferers and their twins (Gilbertson et al. 2002).

The present neuroscientific research era is increasingly linking brain activity with mind experiences via neuroimaging studies. In a positron emission tomography (PET) study of PTSD, patients' brain activity was monitored while they were exposed to previously written vivid narratives of their own traumatic experiences. During exposure subjects demonstrated heightened activity in the right hemisphere only in the limbic areas most involved in emotional arousal. Such activation was also associated with heightened activity in the right visual cortex, reflecting the flashbacks they reported. Most significantly Broca's area – of the left hemisphere, which is responsible for translating personal experiences into communicable language – appeared to switch off. Patients' difficulties putting feelings into words were actually reflected in changes in brain activity (van der Kolk 1996b).

Neurochemistry and PTSD

The basic stress response involves two neurochemical systems: that dependent on corticotrophin-releasing factor (CRF) and the locus ceruleus-autonomic nervous system (LC-ANS) (Staner 2003). Both systems result in hormonal, behavioural and autonomic responses and there is two-way communication between these systems. The LC-ANS is more reactive to physiological stressors, while the CRF system is more relevant to environmental hazards. Danger cues provoke the secretion of brain neuropeptides, which stimulate the paraventricular nucleus of the hypothalamus to release CRF, vasopressin and other neuropeptides (Yehuda 1999). CRF-containing neurons located in the central nucleus of the amygdala activate fear-related behaviour, while inhibiting exploration (Staner 2003). CRF is released into the hypothalamo-hypophysial portal system and transported to the anterior pituitary where it stimulates secretion of adrenocorticotrophic hormone (ACTH), which stimulates the release of glucocorticoids from the adrenal glands (Graham et al. 1999). CRF coordinates behavioural, immunological and autonomic responses of mammals to stress. CRF also mediates the release of noradrenaline from the locus coeruleus, mediating arousal and vigilance. CRF thus is a prime regulator of the stress response. There are two receptor subtypes of CRF. CRF1 mediates ACTH release, while CRF2 regulates emotional behaviour. A major function of cortisol is to contain stress-activated reactions and terminate the HPA stress response by a feedback loop (see Figure 3.2). The HPA in PTSD appears hyper-responsive in some respects but negative feedback inhibition seems to paradoxically produce decreased basal cortisol levels, the opposite of what might be expected for an extreme stress state (Yehuda and McFarlane 1995; Yehuda et al. 1998).

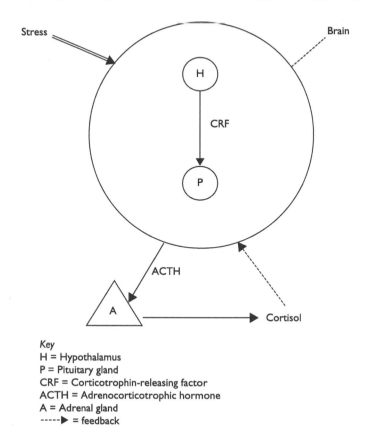

Key
H = Hypothalamus
P = Pituitary gland
CRF = Corticotrophin-releasing factor
ACTH = Adrenocorticotrophic hormone
A = Adrenal gland
-----▶ = feedback

Figure 3.2 The hypothalamo-pituitary axis and stress-related hormonal responses

PTSD involves extreme autonomic responses to stimuli reminiscent of the trauma, loss of ability to discriminate between benign and threatening stimuli and chemical changes including elevated catecholamines, decreased levels of glucocorticoids and serotonin, but increased opioid activity (van der Kolk 1996c). The locus coeruleus in the dorsal pons of the brainstem serves a key noradrenergic function, sending projections to the cerebral cortex, thalamus, hippocampus, amygdala, hypothalamus and other brain sites (Bremner et al. 1999). Serotonin mediates the suppression of behaviours motivated by emergencies or previous reward via the septo-hippocampal system. Endorphins and oxytocin inhibit memory consolidation whereas excessive noradrenergic or vasopressin release at the time of trauma may play a role in the 'excessive' consolidation of trauma memories (van der Kolk 1996c). This is likely to account for the characteristic day-to-day forgetfulness of PTSD sufferers. Reliving traumatic memories may possibly release stress hormones providing a positive feedback loop, possibly causing subclinical PTSD to develop into PTSD.

Chronic stress can result in sustained increases in cortisol or its depletion (with no elevation). For example, laboratory rats exposed to cats for twenty days still show higher basal corticosterone levels suggesting lack of habituation (Blanchard et al. 1998). While major depression is associated with both chronic stress and elevated cortisol levels, PTSD sometimes displays paradoxically decreased levels of cortisol, despite the obvious stress relationship (Yehuda 1999). Women with histories of previous assaults have been found to have lower mean acute cortisol levels after rape but higher probabilities of developing PTSD. These findings were consistent with animal studies demonstrating reductions of HPA responses to stressors after previous exposures to stress (Resnick et al. 1995). Many have considered reduced cortisol levels in PTSD to reflect a chronic PTSD adaptation, assuming that in the acute phase cortisol would have been elevated, but lower cortisol metabolites have been found in Vietnam soldiers under imminent threat of enemy attack (Bourne et al. 1968).

The low cortisol level of PTSD might result from priming a chronic compensatory adaptation of the HPA (De Bellis 2001). Cortisol levels might also reflect the balance between an undifferentiated arousal state of engagement, with higher cortisol levels, and opposing anti-arousal disengagement defence mechanisms such as numbing, with lower cortisol levels. Low cortisol levels in PTSD might be psychogenic, reflecting coping strategies. Hence, cortisol levels cannot be used as markers for PTSD (Mason et al. 2001).

Complex PTSD involving trauma and deviation of the developmental trajectory may share features found in reports in rodents and non-human primates of dysregulation of the HPA axis due to early adverse life events. In rodents these neurobiological alterations have been shown to persist into adulthood (Graham et al. 1999). Early adverse experiences seem to sensitize organisms to stress later in life. Non-human primates allowed visual but not physical access to mothers demonstrated the same behavioural changes observed in abandoned and neglected children (Albeck et al. 1997). Similarly rats, which underwent maternal separation for six hours per day between days 10 and 21 of life, demonstrated persistent alterations in HPA responses to stress in adulthood (Ladd et al. 1996). A study of bonnet macaque monkeys reared under chronic stress showed elevated cerebrospinal fluid CRF concentrations but reduced cerebrospinal cortisol levels identical to findings in PTSD (Coplan et al. 1998).

The catecholamines adrenaline and noradrenaline are excitatory and responsible for physiological arousal. The locus coeruleus is the brain's primary neuronal centre for the ascending dorsal noradrenergic system and can be seen as a trauma centre or central relay station, responding rapidly to incoming information. Located in the pons it innervates areas implicated in significance discrimination, fear and memory formation in the limbic system and cerebral cortex. Stress increases vigilance and enhances memory recall, promoting survival in threatening situations (Bremner et al. 1999).

Inflicting bilateral experimental lesions in the locus coeruleus in monkeys results in their failing to display appropriate fear (Krystal et al. 1989). The locus coeruleus is involved in fear and memory formation in the limbic system and cerebral cortex. It is also the centre for the ascending dorsal noradrenergic system. It primes the organism to detect danger. Noradrenaline is secreted by the locus coeruleus and distributed throughout much of the central nervous system, particularly the neocortex and limbic systems (van der Kolk 1996c). It plays a role in memory consolidation and the initiation of flight or fight behaviours. Release of noradrenaline onto motor neurons via extended lateral amygdala activation of the locus coeruleus may enhance motor performance during fear states (Davis and Whalen 2001).

Serotonin is involved in the regulation and reduction of aggressive behaviour (and many other functions). Decreased serotonin levels have been found in inescapably shocked animals. Selective serotonin reuptake inhibitor (SSRI) antidepressants, which enhance serotonin neurotransmission activity, are helpful for reducing impulsivity and aggression in humans (van der Kolk 1994).

The avoidance symptoms of emotional numbing, decreased interest in activities and feeling detached from others may be related to alterations in mesocortical and mesolimbic dopaminergic systems. Dopamine research in PTSD has been relatively neglected, but the little evidence available suggests there may be increased dopamine activity in PTSD (Bremner et al. 1999). Dopamine is involved in motivating behaviours by rewards, thereby playing a key role in addictions. It also is involved in arousal.

In the Second World War, surgeons working in the battlefields noted that wounded soldiers had a reduced need for opiate analgesic medication (Bremner et al. 1999). Stress-induced opiate-mediated analgesia protects organisms against feeling pain while actively involved in defence (Krystal et al. 1989). Under stress endorphins, noradrenaline and oxytocin are secreted and interfere with storage of experience in conscious memory. They modulate pain, reduce stress and promote calm. Oxytocin in childbirth may contribute to the rapid forgetting of the pain (van der Kolk 1994). Freezing and numbing experiences may allow organisms to not consciously experience or remember situations of overwhelming stress (van der Kolk 1996c).

Conditioning studies and functional anatomy

The conditioning studies described earlier may not tell us all we need to know about emotions and the brain, or even about fear and the brain, but they have been an excellent starting point (LeDoux and Phelps 2000). Fear conditioning can occur via the thalamo-amygdala or thalamo-cortico-amygdala pathways. The former is rapid, subconscious and may prime the latter. Conscious perception is not necessary to activate fear. Fear can be activated by environmental stimuli too weak or peripheral to reach one's conscious awareness (Ohman et al. 2000).

Many of the amygdala's connections are already formed in the adult organism, as electrical stimulation produces fear without prior conditioning. Davis and Whalen (2001) suggest that much of the complex behavioural pattern seen during a state of 'conditioned fear' has already been 'hard wired' during evolution. Fear does not even have to reach the cortex for fear conditioning. Even fruit flies and snails can be conditioned to 'fear' responses. Lesions in the amygdala reduce fear conditioning, emphasizing its importance in this function (LeDoux 2002). As fear conditioning does not necessitate conscious awareness, soldiers may become conditioned to repeated battlefield sounds associated with fearful situations, which they have never considered. Any later extinction of such associations results from the brain controlling fear, not from the elimination of emotional memory. This is suggested by the fact that an extinguished response can be easily reinstated – the memory never went away, it was only suppressed.

The extinction of behavioural responses to aversive memories may occur in the absence of reinforcement. The extinction process involves the basolateral amygdala. Recent research on mice suggests that endogenous cannabinoids (natural neurotransmitters related to cannabis) may be involved in extinction of aversive memories and may be a potential therapeutic target in PTSD, phobias and some forms of chronic pain (Mariscano et al. 2002).

Neurogenesis and plasticity

LeDoux (2002) commented: 'many human mental disorders – including anxiety, phobia, posttraumatic stress syndrome and panic attacks – involve malfunctions in the brain's ability to control fear.' This is the traditional conceptualization of PTSD's basis. An evolutionary model involving adaptation provides a contrasting interpretation. However, both are compatible with observations that PTSD may be associated with lasting neuronal changes in response to stress, with relatively enduring effects on long-term memory as a result of the stress's evolutionary significance. The traditional conceptualization implies the changes serve no function; the evolutionary explanation suggests they may have been adaptive though not necessarily in the present time.

Neuroscientific research points to the shrinkage of the hippocampus in PTSD (van der Kolk 1996c). Most describe this as pathology and I would agree from the individual's perspective. However, there is a possibility that hippocampal shrinkage might have been adaptive in ancestral and possibly even the present time. PTSD involves a tendency to focus on defence-related memories at the expense of the more day-to-day memories. The question arises as to whether hippocampal shrinkage might reflect a reduction in new storage of 'trivial' non-defence-related information making way for new defence-related information receiving priority. It is accepted that under certain circumstances programmes for selective cell death (apoptosis) may operate (Panksepp 1998). Metaphorically, if an office were taken over as a war operations centre, it would be helpful to clear the room of irrelevant materials.

Adult male rats exposed to fox odours, but not to non-threatening odours, experience a rapid decrease in the number of proliferating cells in the dentate gyrus of the hippocampus (Tanapat et al. 2001). This is in keeping with brain changes in humans with PTSD. Experiments with other stressors and other mammals led Tanapat and colleagues (2001) to suggest that regulation of the process involved in such cell proliferation may be a feature of all mammals. However, the fox odour effect on rats was only transient, being detectable at one week but not at three weeks. Is this a problem for the evolutionary theory of PTSD? No, I do not believe so. A component of the theory is that re-experiencing symptoms keeps the memory of the stressor alive and individuals with PTSD remain stressed, implying some ongoing increased HPA activity.

The hippocampus can be seen as the gateway to memory, processing information before it is relayed on from long-term storage in cortical areas. Hippocampal damage results in difficulty learning but the recall of established memories remains intact (Kempermann and Gage 2002). Surgical removal of the hippocampus has little effect on fear conditioning except conditioning to specific contexts, one of the hippocampus's key functions (LeDoux 2002). The amygdala can provide the conditioned fear sensations, but the hippocampus is necessary for entry of contextual information. While conscious memory is selected for storage by the hippocampus, it is the cortex that actually stores it.

Lizards and other lower animals are capable of massive neuronal regeneration following brain damage, but mammals are not (Kempermann and Gage 2002). Generally neurons are generated during restricted developmental periods and the mammalian brain has been considered non-renewable (Rakic 2002). Extensive evidence demonstrates that the foremost exception to this rule in mammals is the dentate gyrus of the hippocampus, the region important for learning and memory (van Praag et al. 2002). Might the hippocampus's capacity for neurogenesis not be functional (Eriksson et al. 1998)? Gould and colleagues (1999) demonstrated that when rats were subjected to learning tasks that involved the hippocampus, the production of adult-generated neurons doubled. In contrast when the learning task did not involve the hippocampus, the production of new cells remained unchanged, suggesting neurogenesis is functional. They suggested that chronic stress may contribute to diminished hippocampal neurogenesis and performance decrements. Van Praag and colleagues (2002) using different methodology have also demonstrated that these new hippocampal neurons are functional.

Summary

The triune brain concept of reptilian, paleomammalian and neo-mammalian development greatly facilitates the understanding of emotional and defence-related aspects of the brain. Despite the concept of the limbic system, there is no brain emotions centre; instead the emotions are organized in a number of modules, separate functional units, including rage/anger, fear/anxiety and panic/separation. Stress triggers the HPA and noradrenergic activation, but the relationship between the two systems is unclear and uncertainties exist regarding the extreme stress response of PTSD. The wiring of structures involved in the recognition of danger and other emotions important for survival relies heavily on older brain structures, with much activity remaining outside of conscious awareness. Older subcortical responses are quicker and may be more relevant for immediate threats. Much of the subjective experience of traumas generating PTSD, and their subsequent re-emergence as symptoms of PTSD, relate to these older brain processes. Hence much of the PTSD experience lies outside of awareness, with flashes of awareness disconnected from coherent associations being one of the major challenges of the condition. Research since the early 1990s or so has provided much of the current knowledge about brain functioning. Conditioning studies can now be integrated with brain studies. Psychiatry's fascination with emotions, such as fear, has been at the expense of context and behavioural function. Greater attention to the concept of vigilance is needed. The finding that the hippocampus, so central to emotional and spatial learning, is the leading brain region with some capacity for ongoing neuronal development as well as loss, begs the question as to whether this might reflect brain adaptation as opposed to purposeless pathology.

INDELIBLE MEMORIES, FORGETFULNESS AND DEFENCE

> Nothing fixes a thing so intensely in the memory as the wish to forget it.
>
> Michel de Montaigne, 1533–1593

The evolution of memory and awareness

Memory is a vital component of learning and therefore vital for defence. Even primitive species would fall by the evolutionary wayside if they did not have the capacity for remembering the negative and positive aspects of their environment. Key evolutionary defence issues include an innate readiness to fear predators, which is complimented by learning. When a predator is recognized as dangerous, it is important to retain memories such as what, when and where. Genetically facilitated learning (preparedness) assists such acquisition of fear responses. Fear of reptiles constituted the prototype, as early reptiles were the dominant predation threat in the paleomammalian era. Disproportionate snake fears have persisted into contemporary times, even in countries where snakes do not exist. Snake fear may be a prototype, but even this requires learning, as we saw in conditioning studies above. It is near universal in the wild but generally absent in laboratory-reared animals (Ohman et al. 1985).

Accurate recall for the imitation of action is present from the first year of human life, well before language develops (Toth and Cicchetti 1998). This cognitive peculiarity fades into insignificance when one considers that unicellular organisms without a nervous system may learn to withdraw from danger (Marks 1987). Further, ants and bees are able to learn complex social behaviours. Memory is not dependent on awareness. However, the pictures in our minds that we call 'memories' involve awareness, and language makes communication of our memories to others much easier. Awareness is completely absent in unicellular organisms and probably minimal in reptiles. An affective awareness is present in all mammals, with cognitive awareness emerging in primates. Self-awareness is probably present in the great apes, but awareness of awareness may be confined to humans (Panksepp 1998). The human self emerges in the second year of life, which sees the start of autobiographical memories. However, most human memories lie outside of our awareness – for example, which muscles would you activate and with how much tension to leave the room?

State-dependent memory and memory laws

All of us contain within our heads vast reservoirs of memories. If they were all simultaneously recalled, we would be overwhelmed. How does the brain know when to retrieve which memories? It would be advantageous if the brain recalled memories relevant to the current environmental challenge. Memory is determined by factors other than actual experience. Where emotion is irrelevant to the material being learned, its presence adversely affects memory, but emotion enhances memory if it is relevant to the cause of the arousal (Toth and Cicchetti 1998). Emotional states have great capacity to influence recall, especially with the passage of time. Concentration camp survivors may have great confidence in their memories but these have been found to change over time. Both pleasant and unpleasant (i.e. affectively influenced) thoughts are more difficult to remember in the short term, but in the long term both are better recalled than neutral thoughts (Searleman and Herrman 1994).

The theory of state-dependent memory suggests that recall will be more accurate when the state of recall matches the state of memory encoding (Searleman and Herrman 1994). The re-emergence of PTSD after decades in remission may occur in war veterans following hospitalization, leading to the re-experiencing of earlier traumatic memories of injuries (Aarts and Op den Velde 1996). Retirement with its multitude of losses, including the distraction provided by employment, may result in late-onset PTSD (MacLeod 1994). The loss of ageing friends may resonate with the earlier loss of fallen comrades.

Trauma interferes with conscious memory, but does not inhibit unconscious memory, which controls conditioned emotional responses, skills, habits and sensorimotor sensations related to defensive experience (van der Kolk 1994). High arousal promotes the retrieval of traumatic memories – both sensory information and behaviours associated with previous trauma. A century ago the Yerkes-Dodson Law of 1908 stated that first, optimal performance is associated with moderate levels of arousal or motivation; and second, higher levels of arousal or motivation are associated with better performance for easy tasks, but worse for difficult ones (Yerkes and Dodson 1908). Higher arousal associated with incentives improves short- and long-term memory, while arousal associated with anxiety decreases both (Searleman and Herrman 1994).

At a brain level the more significance the amygdala assigns to memories, the more they will be retained. However, very high levels of arousal may prevent the proper evaluation and categorization of experience by interfering with hippocampal function. This may lead to later retrieval as isolated images, bodily sensations, smells and sounds that feel alien and separate from other life experiences (van der Kolk 1996b).

The Easterbrook Hypothesis (1959) suggested that high states of arousal narrow the focus of attention, decreasing attention to irrelevant cues (Searleman and Herrman 1994). This explains the first assumption of Yerkes-Dodson Law, i.e. that optimal performance is associated with moderate levels of arousal, because at low arousal there are too many irrelevant cues being attended to, but at high levels some important cues become ignored. Walker's (1958) action-decrement theory asserts that high arousal inhibits short-term recall, but consolidates memory, enhancing its recall when arousal later declines (cited in Searleman and Herrman 1994). This is highly relevant to the inability to forget traumatic memories reported by sufferers of PTSD. Hence, there are a multitude of factors influencing what may be recalled.

Fear as a component of a behavioural module

Tooby and Cosmides (2000) described emotions as serving super-ordinate functions to override lesser mental programmes. Fear shifts perception and attention, lowering the threshold for threatening signal detection. During threat assessment goals and motivational weightings change, with safety becoming a higher priority. Information-gathering programmes are redirected to the sources of threat. Conceptual frames shift with the automatic imposition of categories such as 'dangerous' or 'safe'. Memory processes are redirected to new retrieval tasks such as considering an escape route. Communication processes change with activation of signals of alarm or speech paralysis. Specialized inference systems are activated such as assessing the behaviour of the detected threat for selection of the appropriate defence strategy. Specialized learning systems are activated with the possibility of an enduring brain-mediated recalibration (Pitman and Orr 1995). Fear-related experiences are much easier to recall than mundane ones. Autonomic changes redirect blood and energy to vital survival functions. Behavioural decision 'response rules' are activated (Wenegrat 1984). Fight back if the attacker is small; flee or surrender if the attacker is large.

The emotions driving defence are primarily fear and aggression. Clinicians are more familiar with the terms 'anxiety' and 'panic' than that of fear. Panic may be more to do with separation than fear of violence per se, although there is an overlap (Panksepp 1998, 2000).

Anxiety and fear lie on a continuum. General anxiety probably evolved to deal with ill-defined threats (Marks and Nesse 1997). Fear is also more immediate than anxiety.

Many threats trigger specific response strategies that can be viewed as situation-dependent algorithms or behavioural modules (Tooby and Cosmides 2000). Heights induce freezing to prevent falling; bleeding or injury may produce fainting to reduce blood loss. Agoraphobia relates to being out of one's territory, promoting a retreat to it. Trauma evokes fear and avoidance. Social threats evoke responses that promote group acceptance, for example, submission, meekness, gaze aversion and other signals of non-threat.

Module selection will also combine probability with weighted consequences (Tooby and Cosmides 2000). Leaving one's baby at home alone in a cot for the morning would probably result in no harm, but the potential consequences are so grave that 'probably' is unacceptable. Where a number of issues need to be simultaneously assessed, algorithms must assign priorities based on importance, reliability of cues and costs. An internal communication system sends a situation-specific signal to all relevant programmes. Finally, each programme and physiological mechanism must have algorithms that regulate how it responds to each emotional signal – for example, fears that might arise in visually obscure situations may reset auditory thresholds – hearing becomes enhanced.

Fear can be considered at three levels: first, short term – responses involve primarily the coordination of perception and action. For example, freeze and stand back from the snake in the grass. Second, intermediate to lifelong – behavioural strategies that are assisted by learning from past experiences. Avoid walking in long grass. Third, long term – strategies that are stable over generations, as reflected by their presence in the gene pool. For example, the innate fear of snakes that exists even in people in countries devoid of snakes (Ohman et al. 2000; Ohman 1986).

Evolved modules of emotions linked with behavioural responses have also been described as response (or epigenetic) rules (Wenegrat 1984). These are species-related response patterns that can be recruited in the presence of certain environmental stimuli. The resulting behaviour has been described as a 'psychobiological response pattern' (Gilbert 1992). Both relate to basic predetermined plans activated by environmental stimuli in the relevant context.

Special police training insights

In Chapter 2 I noted that unpleasant emotions depend on the activation of an evolutionarily primitive subcortical circuit, including
the amygdala and its neural projections. This mediates specific autonomic and somatic reflexes that originally promoted survival in
dangerous conditions. When subjected to sudden unexpected threat
individuals may react first (e.g. startle), become afraid second, and
only thereafter cognitively appraise the situation. The automacity of
fear is independent of slower, language-based appraisal processes
(Lang et al. 2000).

Most emotional processing is at an unconscious level (Bargh and
Chartrand 1999; Panksepp 1998). Many emotionally driven behavioural responses are too rapid for feelings to have been aroused. A
startle response may take less than one-hundredth of a second. A
person simply cannot think that fast. Thinking follows the emotional
and behavioural responses of startle. 'What was that?' is often the
first cognition that follows the startle response and this very question
illustrates the cognitive delay.

Subjective reports of memories in response to threats are not
available from the animal world. However, useful insights into primitive fear-related memory registration have been studied from a police
training perspective (Artwohl and Christensen 1997). The findings
are useful to review as I am suggesting PTSD can be viewed as
an overactivation of normal defensive states. Fear effects we have
already noted include analgesia whereby those seriously injured may
fight on without registering that they have been injured. Other seemingly unreal dissociative phenomena occur. 'Tunnel vision' involves
loss of peripheral vision, directing full attention at the threat. It is an
asset with a price. It permits rapid reaction to the major source of
threat, for example a pointed gun, but may constrict attention so that
scanning for other threats is inhibited. In contemporary policing this
is known as the 'Weapon Focus Phenomenon' (Loftus et al. 1987;
Searleman and Herrman 1994). Police need to be trained to recognize and respond appropriately to the possibility that while the gun
pointed at them merits close attention, it may not be the only gun
directed their way.

In fear states memories may be 'snapshot' in quality with no coverage of the general environment – lacking the panning sweep shots
of the amateur video camera operator. Animal studies suggest a
shutdown of the prefrontal cortex under fear conditions, as control

is transferred to subcortical defence circuits (Ohman and Mineka 2001). Hence, it is not surprising that years later PTSD memories are full of gaps (Searleman and Herrman 1994).

Studies consistently report that greater emotional arousal leads to inferior memory for peripheral details and vice versa. Artwohl and Christensen (1997) conducted a survey of police responses to life-threatening situations. These bear remarkable similarity to experiences encountered in PTSD. Paradoxical heightened visual clarity for some details but not others has been noted. This might involve having a clear image of an assailant's gun but not being able to recall his face. Hearing distortions may result in shots not being heard at all. Time distortion may involve slow or fast motion time. Dissociation may result in a subjective departure from a state of fear to feeling almost nothing as the focus on survival increases. Temporary paralysis (freezing) may inhibit the firing of weapons in acute encounters. Intrusive thoughts may include thoughts of not seeing one's family again. Automatic behaviour may lead to a police officer shooting a person, only to immediately regret it, and be unable to account for how this happened. Memory gaps and/or distortions may also involve recalling things that never happened.

The following perceptual distortions were reported in a survey of seventy-two police officers involved in deadly force encounters (Artwohl and Christensen 1997): diminished sounds 88 per cent, tunnel vision 82 per cent, automatic behaviour 78 per cent, heightened visual clarity 65 per cent, slow motion time 63 per cent, memory loss for parts of the event 61 per cent, memory loss for some of officers' actions 60 per cent, dissociation 50 per cent, intrusive distracting thoughts 36 per cent, memory distortion 19 per cent, intensified sounds 17 per cent, fast motion time 17 per cent and temporary paralysis 11 per cent. Police training emphasizes two kinds of thinking: experiential (high arousal) and rational (low arousal) – the automatic and the considered. The automatic will be faster and subcortically mediated. Special police are encouraged to use fear rather than resist it. Stress inoculation training is employed in police training. It consists of conceptualization of the stressor, skills acquisition, rehearsal and application and follow through. Repetitive training is required in part to activate rapid reptilian responses. These police research insights vividly demonstrate cognitive fragmentation and also demonstrate that acute fear responses are remarkably similar to the experiences reported by those with PTSD.

Emotions as communicational states

Emotions serve both social and non-social survival functions. However, in neomammalian social evolution, emotions drove the rapid development of another function – that of communication. While social evolution may have driven language, language may also have driven social evolution. Both are associated with neocortical expansion. Human language is associated with complex social interactions and social systems. The social communication functions of human emotions are sufficiently complex that much of human psychopathology may be viewed as based on social physiology (Gardner and Wilson 2004). Depression reflects submissive and other such communications; anxiety states communicate danger; paranoid states communicate aggression (Stevens and Price 1996).

Emotions serve their dual motivational and communicational functions concurrently and inseparably. Social bonding is associated with both feelings motivating closeness and signals that closeness is safe and desirable. An approach/avoidance conceptualization to the functions of emotions is useful. PTSD tends to relate more to the latter.

While the human capacity for logic is impressive, we arrogantly overstate the extent of its development. Looking back in evolutionary time we have no challenger. Looking forwards, we have a long way to go. Logic is generally thought to be factual. Our perception of facts in reality becomes heavily influenced by emotions. This is at the heart of the confusing subjective experience of most psychiatric disorders – especially PTSD. PTSD involves not only conspecific issues similar to those seen in affective disorders, but also predation-related phenomena.

Information processing and PTSD

Information-processing models of PTSD drew on work of cognitive behaviourists. Ohman et al. (1985) presented an information-processing model involving, first, automatic processing, which is unconscious, rapid, effortless, non-analytical, and reflects overlearning routinized processing acts. Military training facilitates this. Soldiers are trained through repetitive exercises to respond automatically to commands or threats. A soldier trained to attack in the presence of certain cues may later with PTSD be prone to respond to those cues in the absence of genuine threats. Second is controlled processing, which is conscious, volitional, slow, sequential, analytical, effort-demanding and creative. Although automatic processing delivers information to the controlled processing system, the systems are independent.

In phobias the automatic processing system overrides the controlled. Phobias may occur in the three systems described by Mayr (1974): non-communicative behaviour is directed at the physical aspects of the environment, e.g. a phobia of elevators; communicative behaviour may be interspecific, e.g. predator defence, producing animal phobias; and intraspecific, producing social phobias.

Chemtob et al. (1988) suggested that traumatized individuals with PTSD experience persistently activated threat-related arousal. Threat-related arousal has potential for threat-seeking behaviour and via a feedback process may fuel re-experiencing phenomena and the generalization of fear.

A female patient of mine who had been attacked during an armed hold-up developed extreme hypervigilance to such an extent that a late appointment with me left her afraid of venturing 20 metres to her car in the now dark on-site car park. With embarrassment she asked my secretary if she would accompany her to her car. Yet that same patient, on another occasion in a safe public venue, aggressively confronted an innocent by-stander with, 'Who do you think you are fucking staring at?' This was quite uncharacteristic of her former self and reinforced the notion that she could not handle public areas. It also paradoxically put her at greater risk of being re-attacked.

Eye contact is usually a threatening signal in the animal world. Although culture has largely offset this in many human cultures, when our biology is in overdrive, as in PTSD, a simple innocent look may provoke hostility.

The information-processing model suggests that fear structures in memory contain information about the feared stimulus, including cognitive, physiological and behavioural responses. Victims of sexual assaults may respond to subsequent unwanted sexual advances quite differently from non-traumatized persons. They may both overreact and paradoxically underreact, giving submissive signals that may put them at risk.

There are three critical information-processing problems in PTSD. First, there is overinterpretation of current stimuli as reminders of the trauma. For example, rowdy diners in a restaurant may reactivate memories associated with a bank robber shouting instructions at a bank-teller. Second, there is generalized hyperarousal, which impairs stimulus discrimination. Hyperarousal creates a vicious cycle involving state-dependent memory retrieval accessing traumatic memories, which consolidate the arousal. In response, the teller in the restaurant scene has to make more effort than his companions to attend to ordinary conversations. Third, there may be dissociation in response to traumatic memories and current life stressors (van der Kolk et al. 1996a). The traumatized bank-teller sitting next to the rowdy diners may be bombarded with fragmented images, feelings and other associations of his/her robbery experience.

A central feature of PTSD is a polarization of experience in which victims oscillate or alternate between intense, vivid and painful memories and a pseudo-normality based on avoidance by means of dissociation, repression and social avoidance behaviours (Horowitz 1986; Spiegel et al. 1988). A surplus of traumatic memories contrasts with a deficit of mundane ones.

A veteran peacekeeper from the Somalian conflict described an unusually trauma-free gardening session. He recalled thinking, 'My mind seems to be a blank at the moment . . . I know I'm here, but it's like I'm somewhere else.' His intrusive recollections had settled but left a void. He continued, 'When I'm not consumed by the devils, I feel I go somewhere else . . . I can see everything else around me but I can't touch it . . . everything's hushed.'

Information-processing models at times have not adequately explained emotional numbing. Litz and Gray (2002) have suggested that numbing is not a primary feature of PTSD. They suggest that PTSD involves preferential allocation of attention to threat, and the arousal this process promotes raises the threshold required to respond to non-threatening stimuli. Persons with PTSD frequently can sit in restaurants only if they have their backs to the wall and a clear view of the entrance/exit. Understandably such an 'allocation of attention to threat' would make social chit-chat difficult. However, to suggest that numbing is not a primary symptom, fails to acknowledge the opiate-mediated analgesia observed in some trauma states. Interestingly, 'apprehension' in relation to predator defences in animals has been defined as a motivational state involving reduction in attention to other activities (e.g. foraging) as a result of increasing the allocation of attention to detecting and/or responding to potential predators (Kavaliers and Choleris 2001). This is consistent with PTSD-related exaggerated threat awareness associated with decreased attention to realistically more relevant stimuli.

Many researchers have noted that information-processing theories of PTSD suggest that life-threatening traumas may disrupt a victim's cognitive templates or schemata that represent the outside world as a safe and predictable place – e.g. respectable-looking people are not seen as threats until a person has been attacked by one (e.g. Silove 1998). Predictability and controllability involve commitments to people, institutions and value systems providing a sense of meaning, belonging and protection against threat. Cognitive schemata based on experience allow people to make sense of their arousing experiences and serve as buffers against being overwhelmed. These schemata also act as filters, selecting the relevant perceptual input for further encoding and categorization (van der Kolk et al. 1996a).

Motor-racing drivers may have dreadful accidents in practice sessions, only to get into reserve cars and carry on. Yet lesser motor vehicle accidents commonly cause PTSD in non-professional drivers. What characterizes trauma is highly personal and depends on pre-existing schemata, especially those involving predictability and controllability. Malice contributes to PTSD and might constitute a third key component of such schemata.

If dissociation occurs at the time of the trauma it is more likely to be employed subsequently. Dissociation is particularly prominent in acute stress disorder, which may consolidate the ongoing use of this defensive strategy (Yehuda and McFarlane 1995). Dissociating the experience may be adaptive under some circumstances, for example in repeated child sexual abuse by a parent – 'this is not really happening to me' – but it may mean the child cannot learn from it (van der Kolk 1996b; van der Kolk et al. 1996a). Child sexual abuse tends to lead to the highest rates of amnesia associated with PTSD. Such dissociation may contribute to the repetition compulsion seen in some sexual abuse victims. Time and again they may put themselves in risky social situations that others choose to avoid.

There are three levels of dissociation (van der Kolk et al. 1996a). Primary dissociation involves the splitting of experience into isolated somatosensory elements, which may be recalled as intrusive recollections, nightmares and flashbacks.

Secondary or peri-traumatic dissociation involves a split between the 'observing' and 'experiencing' selves (van der Kolk et al. 1996a). Public-speaking anxiety involves this process. A speaker may in a sense leave herself and become a critical observer. As she does so she may hear her voice falter, which escalates the anxiety with potential for it to escalate out of control. This phenomenon is known as 'spectatoring'. In PTSD the cause may be more profound, such as rape. If the sufferers are not engaged in active interaction with others they may be able to 'tune out', observing their traumatic memories from afar with a lesser sense of experiencing them. Passive interaction, for example complying with unwanted sexual intercourse, whether with a rapist or later with a well-meaning partner, may result in the experience of a variety of feelings of unreality, detachment and confusion.

Tertiary dissociation is more profound. States of self may be constructed that compartmentalize the traumatic emotions, with one state being aware of the trauma and other states being unaware (van der Kolk et al. 1996a). In its most developed form this is known as dissociative identity disorder (DID), formerly called multiple personality. Most sufferers of DID have suffered severe childhood sexual or physical abuse over extended periods. The personality that contains the memory may be stuck at the mental level at which the trauma occurred. 'Daddy's little princess' and sex object may result in a later highly ambivalent adult sexual approach/avoidance orientation.

Child sexual abuse encountered in clinical psychiatric practice often involves very young children – occasionally even babies. This may result in intense emotional states being processed from this developmental mentality.

A patient with DID, whose childhood was extremely traumatic, recurrently asks me in therapy sessions, 'Have I done wrong?', reflecting her expectation of punishment.

Memories of trauma may have no representation in conscious memory. However, physiological arousal may trigger unconscious memory processes of traumatic memories (van der Kolk 1996c). As a result infantile emotional (as opposed to cognitive) memories and adult fears can lay dormant (unconscious and unexpressed) for years until they are reactivated by stress.

Summary

Memory is a prerequisite for survival from the lowest to the highest of organisms. It is awareness of memory that is so variable. Affective states have the power to influence memory storage and recall. Memory will be recalled more reliably when the state in the present time more closely matches the state at which memories were laid down. In survival situations memory becomes focused on survival tasks. Further defence-related states may activate rapid reptilian memory that lies outside of awareness. Police officers under serious threat report acute short-lived symptomatology similar to that seen in acute stress disorder and PTSD. PTSD involves persistently activated threat-related arousal with oscillation between re-experiencing and avoidance of traumatic stimuli. The perception of stimuli involves highly personalized conceptual schemata that greatly influence their traumatic potential. PTSD involves preferential allocation of attention to and overinterpretation of potential threats, hyperarousal and dissociation.

Part II

Evolution and posttraumatic stress disorders

Sit down before fact like a little child, and be prepared to give up every preconceived notion. Follow humbly wherever and to whatever abyss Nature leads, or you shall learn nothing.

Thomas Huxley, 1825–1895

Chapter 4

The evolution of human defensive behaviours

> There are times when fear is good. It must keep its watchful place at the heart's controls. There is advantage in the wisdom won from pain.
>
> Aeschylus, 525–456 BC

ANCESTRAL ORIGINS AND PREDATION PRESSURE

> There is nothing permanent except change.
> Heraclitus, c. 540–470 BC

In the beginning . . .

Let us journey back in time . . .

Approximately 3500 to 2800 million years ago single cell organisms appeared on earth. Multicellular organisms developed 1500 to 600 million years ago – more than half-way through the history of life on earth. Microorganisms dominated the first 85 per cent of life on earth. Multicellularity probably evolved as an 'anti-predator strategy' (Stearns and Hoekstra 2000). Predation pressure – or natural selection involving survival despite predators – has fuelled the development of anti-predator strategies.

Dating the arrival of complex forms of life by fossil or molecular evidence is very imprecise, with little agreement between different writers. I am not inclined to break this tradition in what follows. The first vertebrates were fish, which arose around 500–450 million years ago. 'The age of the fishes' (408–360 million years ago) in the Devonian period was followed by 'The age of the amphibians' (280–248 million years ago). Tetrapods (four-limbed animals) originated about 400–350 million years ago in the form of early amphibians. The first reptiles arrived around 350–280 million years ago (Stearns and Hoekstra 2000).

Just over 230 million years ago in the late Triassic the reptilian lineage gave rise to the dinosaurs and primitive crocodiles. Shortly after, around 230–190 million years ago, mammals evolved from mammal-like reptiles. Hence mammals evolved via primitive fish, amphibians and then reptiles, via many intermediaries (Stearns and Hoekstra 2000). During the Jurassic period dinosaurs were overwhelmingly successful and mammalian development and diversity was minimal, mostly limited to shrew-like creatures. The extinction of the dinosaurs around 65 million years ago may have been caused by a massive meteorite or by more gradual climate change. It resulted in the rapid evolution of mammalian complexity and diversity.

Ancestral forms of various mammalian lineages arose around 65–60 million years ago. These involved rats, mice and squirrels; rabbits and hares; cetaceans (whales, dolphins, etc.); ungulates; and carnivores (Stearns and Hoekstra 2000). The first monkeys appeared about 50 million years ago. The common ancestor of orangutans, the first of the contemporary great apes, branched off from the African apes 13 million years ago, with gorillas branching off 10 million years ago. The common ancestor of chimpanzee and humans lived about 4.9 million years ago. Chimpanzees are more closely related to humans than they are to gorillas. *Homo sapiens* arrived only 150,000 to 230,000 years ago (Wrangham and Peterson 1996).

The human brain is not very adept at numerical perspectives. Hence, let us imagine evolutionary timeframes as distances. Let us call the origin of planet Earth 4550 million years ago as lying 4.55 kilometres from your feet. In which case the following approximate distances are relevant to present considerations:

the arrival of first life on earth	3.5–2.8 **km**
first vertebrates (fish)	500–450 **m**
first reptiles	300 m
first mammals	200 m
last dinosaurs	65 m
first monkeys	50 m
first of present-day great apes (orangutan)	13 m
first bipedal hominids	4 m
first *Homo erectus*	1.6 m

first neanderthal   20 cm
first *Homo sapiens sapiens*   5 cm
first writing (6000 years ago)   6 mm

If the advent of writing is taken as the dawn of civilization, the evolutionary distance, from the first vertebrates, reptiles and mammals whose fundamental characteristics we still share, to the present day is staggering.

Learning and defence

Defence from its most primitive of origins to twenty-first century warfare requires learning. Consider again the above metaphorical distances and that evolutionary theory suggests that there should be continuity from the simplest to the most complex forms of learning. Of sea-dwelling animals, primitive metazoa, e.g. some coelenterates (e.g. jellyfish) and echinoderms (e.g. sea urchins), had greater ability to profit by experience than single celled organisms (Harlow and Meares 1979). Oligochaetes of the phylum annelida (segmented worms) evolved further learning capacity, but did not develop the 'rationality' of cephalopods (e.g. octopus). Teleost fish were still further on.

The advent of land animals (amphibians and reptiles) did not result in any sudden superiority of learning capabilities. In terms of evolutionary leaps, that from protozoa to coelenterates was vast, as the former had no nerve cells, unlike the latter (Marks 1987). A lesser leap to platyhelminthes (flatworms) occurred, which developed the cephalic ganglion. Further, even lesser leaps resulting in the dogfish occurred with more neurons and greater elaboration of the forebrain. The step from dogfish to human was very slight, with that from monkey to human being negligible in comparison. While from a behavioural perspective evolution in its later years has raced ahead, from a morphological perspective the developmental rate has not changed much over the last 200 million years, nor from the birth of life itself.

Organisms at all evolutionary levels face certain common survival problems including avoiding predators, facing dangers from conspecifics, negotiating hostile physical environments, finding food, locating mates, raising young or providing other strategies promoting offspring survival (Plutchik 1980). These behaviours in all but the most basic species have gene-neural mechanisms, which share common origins and are highly prevalent throughout the animal world – present and past.

Common evolutionary misconceptions

One of the most widespread and massive misconceptualizations of evolutionary theory was addressed by Richard Dawkins (1976) in his provocative book, *The Selfish Gene*. He argued persuasively that evolution for the survival of the species is the exception, not the rule. Mostly evolution requires survival of only genes. Genes employ 'gene carriers' for their survival and it is usually helpful for the gene carriers also to survive and reproduce. What is a gene carrier? You and I, for a start. Organisms according to Dawkins can be seen as servants of their genes. If the transmission of genes is facilitated by the organisms carrying them surviving to the next generation, then so be it. At times, however, genetic success may be better promoted if the clumsy gene carrier is dropped. Animals too old for reproduction become prime prey for predators. It is more important that the animals' descendants survive as they can still perpetuate their genes.

The Selfish Gene was a milestone. However, its title reflects other common misconceptions, suggesting that genes can think and personalizing genetic logic. Organic chemistry is not a personal affair. Genetic logic is just that of chemical replication. In its very worst form, confusing human and genetic logic contributed to the eugenics of the Nazi era. Because a phenomenon is favoured by genes, a result of chemistry or nature does not mean it should be tolerated in a civilized society. Such personalized approaches to writing about evolution are technically incorrect but make a more entertaining story.

Behavioural and emotional adaptations reflect ancestral environments (Tooby and Cosmides 1990). Many of our genes are the same as in primitive bacteria, with it being almost certain that those early genes have survived largely unchanged in the journey from unicellularity to *Homo sapiens sapiens*. What modern genes we do possess are mostly those that evolved for Stone Age conditions, with little genetic change of significance occurring since that time.

It is common for comments regarding evolution to become confused by differing timeframes. For example, should a major nuclear war occur, planet Earth may recover quickly from an evolutionary timeframe perspective. This perspective is quite different from that infinitely more relevant to ourselves – a major nuclear war may result in the end of life as *we* know it. The two perspectives should never be confused, but often are.

Beahrs (1990), for example, suggested that traumatized patients should be adversely selected against by evolutionary forces involving 'heightened vulnerability to minor stressors, reckless endangerment, and overt self-destructive actions like substance abuse and suicide . . . [and] reproductive capacity is impaired by difficulty sustaining the intimate relationships'. While this reasoning has some legitimacy, it fails to acknowledge that much of fundamental survival behavioural evolution predated the first hominids. Further, very few significant genetic changes have evolved since the concept of 'patients' was invented. Present conditions and selection pressures are largely irrelevant to the present design of organisms. Contemporary genes will mostly be dated; some will be outdated and destined to fall by the wayside, mostly many generations into the future.

Anatomical and behavioural similarities often point to genetic relatedness. They do not prove it. Chimpanzees and humans have similar morphological characteristics and solve somewhat similar problems, with more similar behaviours than other mammals. It also turns out that our genetic DNAs are very similar. We are indeed closely related.

Humming-birds are noted for their ability to flap their wings at amazing speed, while hovering stationarily in the air just beyond flowers; the birds require amazingly long tongues, if they are to obtain the nectar. No perch is provided by the plant that would make it easier for birds to approach it. Humming-bird hawk moths do exactly the same. One is a bird; the other is an insect. Their similarities are known as 'homoplasy' (Stearns and Hoekstra 2000). Their evolutionary 'convergence' is due to the challenge presented, not due to genetic similarity. There is great potential for a naive attribution of all morphological and behavioural similarities to genetic relatedness. Convergence must always be considered as an alternative explanation, especially where there is little potential for alternative solutions to the environmental problem posed.

Another common error is to fail to differentiate between potential capability and achievement. Consider a fledgling bird a few days before and after learning to fly (Harlow and Meares 1979). Consider also the achievements of 'primitive' Amazonian tribes in the twenty-first century versus the achievements of those in the developed world. Genetically we are almost identical. Similarly, the achievements of

Homo sapiens are disproportionate to other primates, largely because of language and culture. There is no evidence of any intellectual gulf between monkeys and humans any more than there is from monkeys to their closest kin below.

Summary

The evolutionary journey from unicellular organisms to modern humans has followed a genetic pathway reflecting all intermediate stages. Characteristics and the genes shaping them have been preserved over many millions of years. Genes and characteristics important for survival are those most likely to be preserved. Common survival problems including defence, especially against predators, will be reflected in contemporary gene-neural mechanisms. Human achievements create an illusion of massively superior genes. Evolution has no end point, only points in time at which successful species will have achieved a closer genetic equilibrium with recent environmental challenges. Such 'recency' is measured in thousands to millions of years, a timeframe of which we are unfamiliar. Human achievements in the recent millennia bear minimal relationship to genetic changes during this period.

REPTILIAN AND MAMMALIAN DEFENCES

> Nature is just enough; but men and women must comprehend and accept her suggestions.
>
> Antoinette Brown Blackwell, 1825–1921

Having observed that we have much in common with earlier life forms – even primitive ones – we now turn our attention to the topic of defence as this greatly assists understanding PTSD. First, let us consider the evolution of behaviour in general. There are common behavioural survival problems (Plutchik 1980). Animals need energy. We must breathe oxygen, and consume water and organic matter. Beyond energy acquisition, reproductive behaviour is also essential. All animals perform these behaviours with relatively minor variations because of evolutionary conservatism. Evolutionary conservatism will constrain behaviours fundamental to survival more than behaviours that are not. A leap in the latter is less likely to be fatal.

Beyond energy acquisition and reproduction, another behavioural prerequisite is defence. Without any one of these behaviours, life will cease. Survival behaviours evolved very early in our ancestral history and have persisted through a vast number of generations prior to the advent of *Homo* (Buss 1991). A key point to understand is that much of human survival behaviour will have evolved up to hundreds of millions of years prior to the advent of hominids, about 5 million years ago. Evolutionary conservatism is as relevant to these behaviours as it is to fundamental morphology.

While survival behaviours have much in common across species, there are also dramatic behavioural differences even within the great ape family to which we belong, despite our great genetic similarity (Wrangham and Peterson 1996). Without genetic variation there is no potential for organisms to change substantially over generations. Without genetic variation evolution ceases to exist. However, focusing on commonalities can be very illuminating and frequently I will be seeking your indulgence in this respect.

Predation and defence

Defence can be conveniently approached by way of the three main sources of external threat, namely predators, conspecifics and the environment. Predation pressure was the dominant external threat and evolutionary challenge, prior to the advent of complex and competitive social interactions in later mammalian species – constituting 'conspecific pressure'. Its more recent results have been built around adaptations to predation pressure. A peacock's ornate tail feathers help it compete for mates (a conspecific pressure), but could only follow, not precede, anti-predator adaptations. Predation laid the early foundations of defence.

Successful predation involves at least five stages: detection, identification, approach, subjugation and consumption (Endler 1986). Anti-predation can be viewed in opposition to these elements, each of which is associated with a number of prey defence options. Prey may employ multiple defences in a single encounter. Some defences will operate at more than one stage, for example toxic or distasteful flesh may be signalled by colour (identification) and if the predator does happen to eat the creature (consumption) it will be unlikely to consume the prey's kin, thereby genetic survival even of the deceased prey is promoted.

Reptilian defences

We have seen that modern mammals evolved via intermediaries including early reptiles, with the mammalian divergence occurring around 200 million years ago. The divergence of reptiles and mammals gave rise to many important differences. Nevertheless, fundamental similarities remained – a vertebral column, ribs, four limbs, two eyes, and so on. Paul MacLean's triune brain concept emphasizes the neurodevelopmental division of the human brain according to these eras. At the time of the divergence, virtually all of the earliest mammalian defences would have been those of reptiles. Subsequently, mammals have had 200 million years to develop new ones and shed some old ones, albeit mammalian development was constrained in the age of the dinosaurs – aggressive defence by the predominantly shrew-like mammals would have been of limited value against dinosaurs.

Greene (1994) comprehensively reviewed reptilian anti-predator strategies, identifying sixty separate defensive adaptations. While many reptilian defences are relevant to humans, others are less so. Mammals (and birds) possess aerobic exercise capacities far in excess of those of reptiles. Reptiles typically react to the threat of predation with a hierarchy of responses relating to the relative risks, energetic demands and intrinsic constraints. The same is true of mammals, but the constraints imposed by energy expenditure are more obvious in the energy-limited reptiles.

Reptiles attempt to avoid detection whenever possible. Typically they react to threats first, by blending in with their environment, for example by the use of immobility. Their adaptations for avoiding detection are more diverse than mammals as these adaptations are highly energy efficient. If immobility is insufficient, locomotor escape (flight) may follow. If that fails, non-combative aggressive defences such as bluff may be used. Reptiles engage a predator directly (fight) only as a last resort (Greene 1999). Reptiles also generally are more solitary creatures with limited capacity for group defensive strategies.

Greene (1994) described eight broad reptilian anti-predator mechanisms (encompassing his sixty adaptations): first, *crypsis* – camouflage if you like – is a defence whereby animals resemble aspects of their environment by colouration, shape, posture and even movement. Some small lizards may conduct their movements during periods when the wind is causing their surroundings to move, thereby being less likely to declare themselves. Some snakes have extremely limited vision for static objects, relying heavily on motion to make vision useful. However, even with more sophisticated human eyesight, motion greatly facilitates detection.

Second, because of their limited aerobic capacities, reptiles' use of *locomotor escape* has required augmentation (Greene 1994). Reptiles tend to escape to locations inaccessible to their predators such as gaps in rocks. Interestingly, primates including humans have also relied heavily on this strategy. The shared defences of flight to a sanctuary – refuging – probably involves convergence, as the slow locomotor escape capacity of primates has been a recent development, not one handed down from earlier mammalian and reptilian times. Our capacity to outrun predators is very limited. Retreat up trees or to some other sanctuary was and still is a vital component of our escape potential.

What reptiles lack in speed they make up for in their imaginative array of augmentations for escape – only imagination had nothing to do with their evolution. Reptilian escape may involve adaptations whereby the reptile can run across water or fine sand, climb smooth vertical surfaces, glide or parachute from heights and slip out of a predator's grasp as a result of the extreme fragility of their skin (Greene 1994).

Bluffs and threats, the third defence, involve signals, but differ in terms of consequences if ignored (Greene 1994). Threats may be followed by a consequential attack, but bluffs are 'empty threats'. Reptilian defences may involve an increase in size, as displayed by snakes rearing up menacingly. This also may be used in mammals such as cats whose fur may stand up, creating an illusion of greater size. We humans have a vestige of this in the hairs on our neck standing on end, a good illustration of a useless characteristic taking time to die out, as its negative consequences are very limited. Intention to bite movements, explosive noises, sudden exposure of bright colours and more rarely large fake eyes are other examples of bluffs and threats used by reptiles. All humans are familiar with the use of bluff and threats.

Fourth, *diversion of attack* may involve directing predators' attention either completely or to an expendable portion of the reptile. Tail displays may divert attacks to this sturdy or disposable portion of the body. Geckos' tails may be shed, left behind in a wriggling state to distract predators and provide them with time-consuming meals while the tails' former owners escape. Some snakes may miscarry their young or regurgitate recent meals providing an appetising or repulsive prospect to the predator, either way serving as a distraction (Greene 1994).

Removal of cues activating predator attack reflexes or other responses is a fifth group of defensive strategies. Two classes of stimuli are particularly widespread in eliciting killing behaviour by predators: movement and the showing of a head. Hiding the head and/or keeping still may inhibit the predator's attack reflex, creating an opportunity for escape (Greene 1994). Freezing is frequently reported in PTSD but has not received the research and clinical emphasis it deserves. Freezing fulfils a number of strategic responses in humans, which will be later described. This most primitive reptilian form of freezing may be of considerable use against snakes, which rely heavily on movements to locate their prey before striking, because of their limited sight.

Novelty, startle effects, and aspect diversity, the sixth group, include bizarre movements, strange behaviour, peculiar noises, the sudden appearance of colours or eye-spots and other novelties that may confuse, intimidate and raise uncertainty in predators about the safety of attack (Greene 1994). The mobbing defences of birds and primates reflect a later mammalian interpretation of this strategy reliant on their greater social cooperation. Contemporary humans use this group strategy in the bullring to rescue injured matadors and thrown rodeo-riders. The gaining of a split second may make the difference between escape and becoming a predator's lunch or receiving a fatal goring.

Offensive defence in mammals is a seventh mechanism that is largely dependent on aggressive signalling and attack. Reptiles have a more widespread and diverse selection of mechanisms to choose from. These include distasteful or toxic flesh, odoriferous secretions, biting and spitting (Greene 1994).

Greene's (1994) eighth group of defences involves miscellaneous other *morphological adjuncts* – including turtle shells, hissing vocalizations and rattle tails. Possession of horns would be an example in mammals.

Many individual defensive phenomena involve more than one defence strategy. For example, freezing may involve crypsis, bluff by way of death-feigning (pretending to be dead), giving rise to the prospect of food poisoning (live meat being fresher), stability for threat assessment, removal of the movement attack cue and even having a distraction effect. This borrows from four of the eight broad reptilian defence strategies and has important implications for our later discussion of PTSD. Cryptic aspects of freezing in humans may have ancient reptilian origins; these do not necessarily preclude the elaboration of this defence with very recent cognitive inputs, although it should be noted that cognitive processing is very much slower than reflexive responses. Soldiers picking up an unexpected danger cue may freeze reflexively and then use their training to stay frozen while assessing the threat without disclosing their whereabouts by movement.

In addition, in any one encounter a number of defensive strategies may be employed. I will illustrate this with a relevant personal experience.

I was walking along a bush track considering these issues when a snake slithered across my path. I assure you, I am not using poetic licence; I was actually pondering these very issues when this obliging reptile interacted with the aforementioned clumsy mammal. Within a fraction of a second, I startled, and almost immediately after this froze. Both of these defences were reflexive. Startle occurs too quickly to be anything but. Beyond my startle and the reflexive component of my freezing, fear followed, arriving within a second or so. My startle may have served the function of scaring the snake. I do not know for sure because I have no recollection of the snake before I startled.

Whether my freezing played any role in my staying hidden, having scared the snake into retreating up the bank before it turned in my direction, I cannot say. It certainly did not strike, but as I did not advance it had no need to. However, my freezing did permit easier assessment of threat, which suggested that neither flight nor aggressive defence was necessary. Within a few seconds at a cognitive level I had identified the snake as of no threat. I was able to do so first, by its non-threatening behaviour; second, its colours and size allowed me to identify its species as a yellow-headed whip snake known to be somewhat poisonous, but timid and with very small jaws, making biting a human difficult. Had I not been a twenty-first century *Homo* with a liking for wildlife books, I would still have identified it as the most common snake I encounter in my home range, and one that has never looked like doing me any harm in the past. I walked on bare foot (as I was on the way to a remote beach) in a state of hypervigilance. Tree roots across the path repeatedly resembled snakes in my extended state of heightened alert. About ten minutes later I reached the beach. Only then did my protracted heightened arousal and hypervigilance subside.

Mammalian defences

Marine reptiles and land-based dinosaurs greatly outsized early mammals and so paleomammalian predator defences predominantly involved crypsis, freezing or flight. Aggressive defence in mammals flourished later, after the extinction of the dinosaurs. Here we have something of great interest in the context of PTSD. Although aggressive defence did exist in early reptiles, its then limited value suggests that its evolutionary development or reactivation in later mammalian species would have arisen in more recently developed regions and neurological pathways of the mammalian brain. Neomammalian defences would have been built around older, more primitive, automatic and rapid defences (MacLean 1990; Ohman et al. 1985).

While many authors have discussed mammalian defences, as far as I am aware no one has comprehensively catalogued them, although Blanchard and colleagues (1991) have made a start. This may in part relate to mammals being more difficult subjects to study. They move faster and for longer than reptiles. They use group defences much more frequently, which introduce all sorts of complex interspecific variations due in part to cost–benefit issues which will be addressed in this chapter. They are also prone to alter their behaviours when they become aware of observers. The study of primates in the wild requires the process of habituation, i.e. primates getting used to the presence of the strangest-looking primates they have ever seen; ones who follow them around with note-pads and binoculars, but do not seem worth worrying about.

Isaac Marks produced an invaluable early work on evolution and human anxiety, in his landmark 1987 text, *Fears, Phobias, and Rituals: panic, anxiety, and their disorders*. Much progress in ecological studies of mammalian defences has occurred since then, with a greater emphasis on group strategies, cost–benefit ratios and understanding the context in which defences occur. Further, perhaps because PTSD had been officially recognized for less than a decade, Marks' otherwise progressive and challenging work paid only modest attention to PTSD.

Marks (1987) described four fundamental mammalian defensive strategies: withdrawal, immobility, aggressive defence and appeasement. Within these four broad mammalian defence categories lie many of the sixty mechanisms described by Greene (1994) for reptiles. However, whereas reptiles use an array of specialized morphological defensive attributes such as spines, armour and poisons, mammals rely on these much less, camouflage and horns excepted. Mammals rely more on behavioural defences, which are more limited in number, but are widely distributed throughout mammalian species (Blanchard et al. 1993).

This traditional division of mammalian defence strategies belies a further distinction – that of individual versus group defences. Group defences are widespread in primates, herd animals, dolphins and many others. Two key components of group defences are cooperation and signalling (communication) to conspecifics. Signalling but not cooperation may also be directed at predators. *Homo sapiens* has made considerable use of group strategies in both defence and offence.

Withdrawal

Avoidance, withdrawal, flight and other escape have been viewed as variants of a broader avoidance strategy (Marks 1987). I will later take issue with this suggestion, but for now my task is to present existing research. As with reptiles, the ideal avoidance response is to remain undetected. This may involve staying spatially or temporally away from predators, and cryptic behaviours enabling the mammal to blend in with its surroundings. However, this is a snapshot perspective which fails to acknowledge the costs of remaining hidden, which I will shortly address.

Withdrawal or locomotor escape, both known as flight, may be based on speed alone or may combine speed with an erratic course to deny their pursuer the predictability of direction of attack. Several escape options add to the predators' difficulties (Marks 1987). Antelope and other open grassland large mammals generally have the edge on predators when it comes to speed. They may even boast or advertise this by spectacular leaps into the air, signalling, 'Let's not waste energy on a game of chase, when I am much more likely to win'. Accordingly, predators back off. Predators to be successful often rely on tactics such as group attacks, and preying on frail individuals. In conspecific agonic (competitive) relationships, subordinates (lesser individuals) need to keep a safe distance from dominants who will behave aggressively if they move too far away (Dixon 1998), as does a parent whose toddler is straying in the direction of the road. This requires the subordinate to keep the dominant in view. Sure enough, toddlers will often fret if they cannot see their dominant parents.

Arrested flight may occur when a threatened individual cannot escape. It comprises behavioural cut-offs, for example, an animal that cannot run away may avert its gaze, close its eyes or adopt cryptic postures – signalling lack of threat and lack of overt surveillance (Dixon 1998). An individual in suburban life confronted with a vicious-looking dog would be wise to avert his gaze (signalling lack of threat) but most unwise to raise his arms, the movement of which may activate the dog's attack response. Arrested flight curiously may be associated with analgesia (decreased pain perception), about which more will be said later.

Immobility

Immobility strategies are twofold – attentive and tonic (Marks 1987). Attentive immobility involves vigilant monitoring of the threat, with preparedness to flee or fight. My freezing in front of the snake was an example of this. In contrast to the emphasis on vigilance in attentive immobility, tonic immobility involves a sudden onset of prolonged stillness with a lesser vigilance component. It is an extreme fear reaction often referred to as being 'scared stiff'. Many predators are reluctant to eat dead meat as it may cause illness. Sudden recovery and rapid flight may follow tonic immobility. In rare instances fatal cardiac arrhythmias may occur (Marks 1987). Although not a mammal, tonic immobility in chickens involves getting literally stuck in an immobile posture for an extended period – the Todesstellreflex (Dixon 1998). This state of immobility is also known clinically as catalepsy and occasionally occurs in humans, particularly in persons using cannabis or suffering schizophrenia. Immobility may serve at least five different defensive functions: crypsis, pausing to assess the danger, signal preparedness to stand one's ground, or conversely signal not being a threat, or suggest disease risk to predators.

Physiological differences occur in attentive and tonic strategies. Motor reactivity tends to be marked in attentive immobility, but almost absent in tonic immobility. Attentive immobility may be more relevant to distant dangers, whereas tonic immobility may be a terminal reaction to being caught (Marks 1987). A prey animal may freeze when it sees a predator in the distance. Carefully watching it from a still posture may prevent detection by the predator. However, if the predator is already on top of the prey, laying still to inhibit its attack reflex and feign being a risk for food poisoning may be a last defensive resort. Experimental infliction of hippocampal, fornical or septal brain lesions increase tonic immobility but decrease attentive immobility in rabbits and rats, whereas cingulate lesions have the reverse effect. From ecological and neurodevelopmental perspectives these different forms of immobility have little in common except the immobility.

Rape victims often report a paralysed but conscious state involving tonic immobility. Police and soldiers in battle may fail to fire their weapons in the presence of the enemy. Of those that do fire, some will have involuntarily frozen first to assess the threat – more consistent with attentive immobility. Immobility may also involve an inability to move or call out.

Aggressive defence

Aggressive defence by prey usually comes into play when a predator is close to seizing its victims (Marks 1987). Being cornered or in possession of young, with limited potential for flight, will tend to activate this strategy. It may entail use of weapons, such as horns or firearms. In social species cooperation with conspecifics may occur, for example mobbing attacks by primates on predators. Chimpanzees and humans have been known to scare off lions in this way.

A subset of this aggressive defence is threat display. Threat postures commonly involve the animal primed to flee or fight; options are open. Ambivalent responses reflect approach/avoidance tensions and uncertainties. Animals scratching or grooming themselves often signal this. Humans also do this, for example fiddling with rings or sweeping one's hair back when in socially intimidating situations (Dixon 1998).

Threat displays may involve bluff, but even bluff may involve reality, a preparedness to use the advertised threat – mirrored in human weapons of mass destruction. Conservation of resources and avoiding risk of injury is generally preferred – long may this prevail. Threat displays may involve one species mimicking another harmful species. In primates and humans, posture and staring may communicate threat – the New Zealand Maori Haka, an intimidating battle challenge, prior to attack or on the rugby field, uses this strategy. Predation drives the evolution of anti-predator aggression both by the deaths of prey less able to defend themselves, and by rewarding fierce defensive reactions by prey, even if this involves bluff. Hence, the prospect as opposed to the reality of being eaten may drive evolution and be of similar relevance to actually being eaten (Stanford 1998).

Appeasement

Appeasement, or pacification by way of negotiation and concessions, is a further strategy that is mostly confined to use with conspecifics (Marks 1987). Submission is the usual response to down hierarchy threats. It both reduces aggression and maintains proximity (Dixon 1998). In primates and humans a noisy and apparently paradoxical return by the defeated subordinate to the dominant may occur. It may signal, 'OK, I'll do what you want if you will have me back.' This strategy depends on the balance of disadvantage associated with defeat resulting in marginalization versus the risk of return. Following a defeat or other put-downs from dominant individuals, subordinates may need to secure their ongoing membership of the group. Dominants of non-human species may comfort vanquished and distressed subordinates seemingly to quell the disturbance.

Body language alone may be sufficient at times to signal submission. Having made a humiliating social gaffe, it is difficult not to avert one's eyes. Diversion or deflection of attack may be considered a subset of appeasement breaking the rule by being useful between species. Leaving a vulnerable group member to the predator, or abandoning a mortally injured soldier to the enemy, may allow the majority of individuals to escape. However, the obligations inherent in reciprocal altruism will tend to deter this strategy, leaving its use for extreme circumstances. Reciprocal altruism is an important concept involving indebtedness through trading favours (Trivers 1985). It requires the maintenance of relatedness, without which there would be no need to return the favour.

Adaptive conservatism and evolutionarily stable strategies

The term 'adaptive conservatism' in this context refers to interactions with unfamiliar animals triggering automatic fear/wariness (Mineka 1992). I consider it so important that I routinely explain this principle to patients with PTSD. Simply put, when in situations of ambiguous threats, defensive instincts suggest it is better to play safe than to be sorry. Its inverse entails risk-taking. The better-safe-than-sorry principle is fundamental to day-to-day struggles with PTSD, explaining why sufferers habitually tend to assume the worst.

Generally the more vulnerable the individual, the sooner this strategy will be employed. Observations of baboons illustrate the often greater adaptive conservatism among females. Both sexes relish meat, but males have developed better hunting techniques. Females under observation in the wild were never seen to join the consumption of a carcass until it was brought back to the troop, or the troop could be clearly seen. They were among the first to leave if the troop moved off, even when there was still meat left to eat. Lone females are of smaller stature and so at greater risk (Strum and Mitchell 1987). However, it is not as simple as you might expect. Pregnant females may take more risks than non-pregnant females and even fit males. Again, I will have to elaborate later to avoid a major diversion. For now, please remember these strategies are generalizations that vary according to contexts.

This 'better-safe-than-sorry' orientation is also an example of what Maynard Smith (1982) described as an 'evolutionarily stable strategy'. Evolutionarily stable strategies are pre-programmed behavioural policies, which have achieved a stable equilibrium as a result of evolution and the many generations involved. Another example is that generally defenders of their homes are more strongly motivated to defend their territory than a conspecific intruder is motivated to take it. This principle was highly relevant to the outcome of the Vietnam War. If this principle were not the case, over evolutionary time chaos would result, as selection would favour intruders. Victorious intruders would then tend to become vanquished territory defenders – an evolutionarily unstable situation.

In the context of predator detection and response to them by prey, the better-safe-than-sorry strategy is both an example of an evolutionary stable strategy and of adaptive conservatism. The cost of failing to identify predators is generally greater than the cost (even adjusted for frequency) of wasted efforts in responding to non-dangerous situations.

Summary

Our ancestral history involved early reptile-like creatures that gave rise not only to modern reptiles but also to the earliest mammals. Human survival functions including defence will reflect both mammalian evolution and our earlier reptilian heritage. Reptilian defences rely more on structural, reflexive and low energy behaviours. Mammals' superior energy capacities permitted greater development of energy-demanding defences, including flight and aggressive defence. Single defensive behaviours may serve multiple strategic functions and be driven by different neurodevelopmental processes. The sociability of many mammalian species permitted the evolution of group defence strategies. Appeasement in particular reflects the group emphasis of mammals, and is mostly an intraspecific defence. Cost–benefit considerations have resulted in a better-safe-than-sorry defensive tendency.

PREDATOR AVOIDANCE, ANTI-PREDATOR STRATEGIES AND FORAGING

> Nature does nothing uselessly.
> Aristotle, 384–322 BC

The functions of emotions

> If the act of procreation were neither the outcome of a desire nor accompanied by feelings of pleasure, but a matter to be decided on the basis of purely rational considerations, is it likely the human race would still exist?
> Arthur Schopenhauer, 1788–1860

The clinical focus of mental health has involved a disproportionate interest in emotions, especially anxiety and depression. Patients are required to talk about their feelings. Emotions seem at the heart of their problems. However, emotions are mere intermediaries motivating appropriate behavioural responses such as approach or avoidance. Relevant emotion without behaviour is of no use, but relevant behaviour without emotion is fine. Insects and other simple organisms have done very well without emotions. Ethologists, studying animal behaviour, find behaviours to be easier to observe than emotions and as they determine various outcomes such as defeat or victory to be of more interest.

Ohman and colleagues (2000) suggest: 'Emotions can be understood as clever means shaped by evolution to make us do what our ancestors had to do to successfully to pass genes on to coming generations.' They constitute response patterns shaped by natural selection to offer selective advantages in certain situations. Each emotion is a programme for accomplishing a specific fitness task, such as attract or attack. Emotions also serve signalling functions. Evolutionarily relevant threat stimuli are highly effective in engaging attention. Hence, emotions fulfil a dual function of driving particular behavioural programmes, while concurrently serving signalling functions (Gardner and Wilson 2004).

Where emotions appear to override reason, directing individuals into seemingly pointless activity, for example grieving, one should consider the possible long-term modification of psychological architecture. The loss of offspring to a predator motivates greater future caution through the pain of loss and grief (Tooby and Cosmides 2000).

Where immediate danger is involved, time is critical and rapid responses may be needed. Here we find there are unclear boundaries between emotion, motivation and behaviour. Consider startle and freezing responses. I have said that emotion may drive behaviours. However, the speed of the startle reaction is such that behaviour occurs prior to the conscious registration of emotion. This also applies to the initiation of attentive immobility, which activates freezing before emotions motivating behaviour according to context-dependent defensive strategies.

It is curious that human attackers of humans tend to be described as angry and aggressive, but animal attackers of humans, only as aggressive (McGuire and Troisi 1998). Yet 'fear' is a word common to the two victim perspectives. A human who has escaped predatory or environmental threats may feel elation, but escaping a conspecific is often associated with the feeling of humiliation. Hence, fear or its aftermath, horror, takes on different appearances depending on the contexts and associated behaviours.

The ecology of threats

> If the immediate and direct purpose of our life is not suffering then our existence is the most ill-adapted to its purpose in the world: for it is absurd to suppose that the endless affliction of which the world is everywhere full, and which arises out of the need and distress pertaining essentially to life, should be purposeless and purely accidental. Each individual misfortune, to be sure, seems an exceptional occurrence; but misfortune in general is the rule.
>
> Arthur Schopenhauer, 1788–1860

Schopenhauer's philosophy centred on the nature of the 'will' being to strive to live in environments of inevitable adversity. Modern life makes this sound an overstatement. However, those living in impoverished parts of Africa nowadays and our ancestors globally face or faced environments very different from our own. Primatologist Craig Stanford (1998) has observed, 'Every wild primate dies after living a life of near-constant peril.' Our wonderful experiment called civilization creates an illusion of contentedness as the normal state, and discontentedness, including anxiety, as being abnormal. While personally I am all for contentedness and the rights of individuals to live without unreasonable levels of anxiety, nature does not share this ideal. In nature, animals face threats from predators, conspecifics, the physical environment, internal and external parasites, bacterial and viral infections, and toxins associated with food (Kavaliers and Choleris 2001). Few failures are as unforgiving as the failure to avoid a predator (Lima and Dill 1990). Predation pressure has played a major role in shaping the gene pool throughout evolution (Ohman 1986; Treves 2002).

Predation is likely to have been the strongest selection factor shaping contemporary anxiety problems. Environments may be dangerous with risks of falls, fires, and others, but these threats are usually highly predictable. Most of the time animals can conclude that their present environmental situation is safe. If this is not the case, they may seek safety by, for example, removing themselves from the risk of falling from a doubtful-looking branch. Risks from conspecifics are substantial but again relatively predictable, permitting a sense of safety much of the time. Safety assessments in relation to predators are less predictable. Predators hide and approach stealthily. Also, they may be more likely to be encountered at a water hole, which is avoidable only for limited periods.

Influences of predation

Studies of birds, mammals and fish have shown that responses of prey to predators are both innate and learnt (Kavaliers and Choleris 2001). The genetic component may produce a basic defensive response, which is then improved by experience. Learning itself is partly genetically controlled.

Anti-predation strategies can be approached via a four-stage model involving the sequence: first, avoidance; second, the recognition or detection phase; third, the pursuit or escape phase; and finally, the subjugation or resistance phase (Vermeij 1982). Predator avoidance and anti-predator mechanisms (within the visual field of the predator) are under different selection regimes and the evolution of one type of prey survival mechanism reduces selection on the other (Brodie et al. 1991). What this means is that the more successful a prey animal is in keeping well away from predators, the less that animal has to bother with defence strategies that might be employed in a distant or close encounter with a predator. Genes will both drive and reflect this. We will later see that this very strongly suggests different genes for different components of PTSD.

Unsuccessful predation is needed for the evolution of anti-predator characteristics, because if all attacks were successful there would only be scope for selection by observation of others. Prey animal A watches B being killed by the predator. B no longer exists, but possibly A may have learnt something useful. An expensive lesson from B's perspective. In reality B often escapes and learns from the experience. Predation promotes evolutionary changes in prey species and such changes may promote further improvements in the predators' strategies. If prey get it wrong, the result is fatal and their genes loosely associated with getting it wrong (except those remaining in kin) are removed from the game of life. Getting it wrong for a predator means it has just missed a meal, so the selection pressure is correspondingly less (Vermeij 1982). Hence, selection pressure favours prey, refining their genes for defence ahead of those of predators.

'Game theory' (a mathematical term) translates well to evolutionary scenarios and permits reducing much behaviour to mathematical equations when considered from an ecological perspective (Mealey 2000). Behavioural defence systems are under extraordinarily strong selection pressure (Blanchard et al. 1998). This prey/predator selection issue just discussed is another example of Maynard Smith's (1982) evolutionarily stable strategies. Evolutionarily stable strategies played repeatedly over evolutionary time cannot be outperformed by alternative strategies (Mealey 2000). If over evolutionary time predators were consistently favoured more than prey by this 'game', it would tend to result in no prey – therefore no predators and no game.

Vigilance, prey decision-making and activity

Vigilance is one of the key concepts of this book, as reflected in the title. I believe mental health researchers and practitioners have much to learn from it. It even gives rise to simple experimentally verifiable new treatment ideas (covered in later chapters). Accordingly, I deal with it in some detail.

Parents teaching their adolescents to drive know that teaching accident avoidance is preferable to teaching them skid correction. Might predator avoidance, as opposed to other more confrontational defences, routinely be the way to go? Life is not so simple. Predator avoidance at times may cost too much. Predator avoidance may be spatial or temporal – avoiding the water hole visited by lions, or going at off-peak times (Brodie et al. 1991). Avoidance limits times or places for feeding, reproducing and raising young (Vermeij 1982; Lima and Dill 1990; Lima 1998). Many people assume that birds will fly off on spotting predators, but this assumption is incorrect. Next time your cat stalks a bird, watch a while. The bird watches the cat, as if thinking, 'Is the effort of flight really necessary?' Birds tend to take flight only when the cat comes close to striking range. Fleeing is costly in foraging time and energy (Proctor et al. 2001).

Lima (1995) studied sparrows' responses to departures from their flocks of other individuals. 'Non-detectors' were sparrows that did not directly detect threats or initiate departure without influence from other flock members. Non-detectors were influenced to flee by multiple departures over a short time interval, with the number of departures being more influential than the proportion of flock departing. Non-detectors were also more influenced by departures originating from the periphery of the group where birds would be more vulnerable to predators and have a better view of them.

Birds are able to detect approaching predators even when not overtly vigilant. However, birds' detection ability was found to be greater when they raised their heads, but this entailed the cost of interrupting feeding (Lima and Bednekoff 1999a). Flocks of birds or herds of animals benefit from the vigilance of others and the time saved may be devoted to foraging. If animals feed close together, competition increases and feeding rates decrease. If individuals space themselves widely, there may be more grass to go round but vigilance efficiency decreases and so predation risk rises. Also assuming predators kill only one victim, animals benefit from the proximity of others by dilution of risk (Proctor and Broom 2000). Many studies have examined these issues in both mammals and birds (Lima and Dill 1990). Sentinels, individuals on the lookout for others, are often observed in family-based groups of birds and mammals.

In the natural world, starvation has been a major selection pressure acting in tandem with predation. However, there is another factor. Our ability to grasp numerically large orders of magnitude is poor. Currently medical researchers are concerned that the golden days of antibiotics are over. Simple bacteria are outwitting the world's best scientists and the dollars of the pharmaceutical industry. How do they do it? They do it by having generations that are sufficiently short in time to mutate at a rate that we cannot keep pace with. Simple numbers. Over many generations selection pressures may achieve startling results. Our egocentric single-generation perspective makes this hard to appreciate.

Prey decision-making under the risk of predation allows an animal to manage predator-induced stress (Lima 1998). The use of the word 'decision' in this context requires some qualification. Simple organisms, even bacteria, are often referred to as being able to make decisions. Even in higher forms of life the mechanism operating may be devoid of awareness. If you go out into your garden after dark, you may feel anxious without being able to give a justifiable account for this.

> You know these things as thoughts, but your thoughts are not your experiences, they are an echo and after-effect of your experiences.
> Friedrich Nietzsche, 1844–1900

Deciding not to feed in the presence of predators may result in energetic stress. An energy-depleted animal may decide that the costs of avoiding or reducing consumption of scarce food because of the presence of predators may be too great and therefore take a calculated risk. The cost-effectiveness of competition for resources will tend to decrease as they are accumulated. While predation pressure may vary little over evolutionary time, over a single lifetime it may vary greatly on a seasonal, daily or smaller timeframe (Lima and Dill 1990).

Even simple animals possess the ability to assess their risk of being preyed upon and incorporate this information into their decision-making. Ants offered a choice of richer or more dilute sugar solution generally chose the richer one, but when placed under predation threat that was greater for the richer solution, they chose the more dilute one. However, when the dilute one was too weak they fed from the richer one despite the predation risk (Nonacs and Dill 1990).

The 'μ/g rule' states that an animal may maximize its fitness, or optimally manage its predator-induced stress, by selecting the behavioural option that minimizes the rate of mortality per unit increase in growth rate (Lima 1998). While there are definite limitations to this concept, the notion that animals may incorporate such a concept into their decision-making process is useful. An energy-depleted animal may be wise to take the time to consume a large meal even though this impacts on predator avoidance. However, an energy-replete animal has less need to take this risk.

In many species a decrease in prey activity tends to follow a period of heightened threat of predation (Lima 1998). Decreased movement and/or increased refuging in response to predation risk occurs in almost all species studied. However, decreased activity may also be associated with increased food availability. Increased availability of food may also attract predators, increasing the risk to prey. Hence, both the threat of predators and an absence of hunger may make it preferable to stay at home. Conversely increased activity, and with it an increased exposure to predators, is associated with energy-stressed animals. A similar cost–benefit analysis determines when prey resume feeding. Lima and Bednekoff (1999b) proposed a 'risk allocation hypothesis' which suggests that animals feeding under time-related variation in the risk of predation, endeavour to achieve optimal anti-predator behaviour across various states of risk. If the risk is high, a defensive orientation is expected, but if the period of high risk is prolonged, the avoidance of feeding over long periods might warrant an adjustment of anti-predator defensive behaviour to compensate for risks associated with energy depletion.

Similarly these issues may influence reproductive behaviour. Females of some species become less choosy with an increase in predation risk (Crowley et al. 1991). (Although we will return to this later, let us stop for a moment and reflect on the possible relevance of the previous sentence for how humans behave sexually in times of war.) Conversely, some species, e.g. some voles, may experience suppression of reproductive activity on exposure to predators.

Costs, benefits and predator-sensitive foraging

Lynne Miller (2002) has described predator-sensitive foraging as representing 'the strategies that animals employ to balance the need to eat against the need to avoid being eaten'. Those who perceive themselves to be less vulnerable to predators exploit riskier settings to increase nutrient intake. She described biological, social and environmental variables. Biological variables are largely or wholly under genetic control. Biological factors promoting safety generally include being a member of a larger or more sexually dimorphic species (where one sex, usually male, is bigger than the other), being an adult as opposed to a juvenile, and being male. Fish, aquatic insects, gastropods, crustaceans, rodents and ungulates have all been demonstrated to be influenced in these respects.

Predator-sensitive decisions may represent adaptive compromises between opposing selective pressures (Miller 2002). Individuals whose fitness is most heavily dependent upon nutrient intake might be expected to take greater risks to access food. Females, despite generally being smaller and more vulnerable in most species, experience greater fitness demands with respect to pregnancy and suckling. These demands may encourage them to take greater risks to access resources. This produces a seeming paradox whereby an individual's physical vulnerability may play a lesser role in foraging decisions than its energetic needs. Remember I suggested just now that larger animals could *afford* to take greater risks. They can, but smaller hungrier ones may *need* to.

Some species favour larger group sizes, others smaller. Large groups decrease time wasted on individual vigilance, which I have already shown reduces feeding time (Lima and Dill 1990). Groups also decrease the risk by providing alternative prey – a dilution of danger to the individual. An increase in group size will increase the area that must be travelled and energy expended to find adequate food supplies (Chapman et al. 1995). However, the major cost of grouping is reduced foraging efficiency.

To emphasize that predator-sensitive foraging is not just some remote notion limited to non- or pre-historic humans, I will take a literary risk by way of a very contemporary illustration. It is not often in modern life that we are directly aware of predation threat and its contingencies. However, living by the beach in Australia I am frequently aware of these issues, as are others who go surfing. Surfers have the potential to become 'shark-bait'. Surf with one friend and your risk of being taken by a shark declines by 50 per cent (the dilution effect). However, the larger the group of surfers, the fewer waves there are to go round (analogous to limited food availability) – the surfer's dilemma.

Interestingly, the fear of being taken by a shark is mostly out of all proportion to the reality. With a few exceptions, the risk of driving to the beach is usually greater than that of being taken by a shark. The disproportionate fear is largely innate, like the fear of snakes. Snakes and predators have been written into our genetic book of life as preparedness. Motorcars have not. We will return to surfing later.

Let us now consider some other biological variables that influence foraging decisions. There are those that are fixed over the lifetime, for example the sensory organs that permit predator detection. There are factors that change slowly, for example increasing body size and ability to defend oneself with maturation. Pregnancy would be another. There are also those that change quickly, for example hunger. These variables influence both vulnerability and incentive to feed; two states that often generate opposing needs (Miller 2002).

I have already touched on some of Miller's (2002) social variables – i.e. larger groups often being safer. Larger groups, because of lower vulnerability, may be able to tap riskier areas. The safest place in a shoal of fish with respect to predation is at the centre. However, energy-depleted fish may do better at the periphery where there are better feeding opportunities. Proximity to others, central positioning in groups and relatedness all reduce danger. Relatedness increases the motivation to defend others because of shared genes and/or reciprocal altruism.

However, proximity to others may reduce foraging success. Group composition would also be expected to influence individual vulnerability. Female gorillas benefit from the protection of massive silverback males and can enter riskier territory as a result. Dare I say it? Desperate prostitutes may be more inclined to risk the seedier parts of town when accompanied by their pimps. Another twenty-first century illustration!

Let us return to the surfer's dilemma. An anxious or vulnerable individual might do well to surf with a *large group* of *close* friends (genetically related family would be even better) and to stay in the *middle* of them. Three separate protective variables are involved here. The surfer's dilemma as we have seen is that he/she may not catch many waves, which reduces the fun of going surfing. When the surfer gets sufficiently frustrated with not getting a wave, he/she may choose to take a risk and move to the edge of, or away from the group where there is less competition, but in the process exposes him/ herself to greater risk of predation. Social rank also may affect foraging. The 'pro-surfer' (professional) may get more waves both because he/she is *more capable* and because he/she commands *respect*. As does the silverback gorilla.

Environmental variables include open areas as opposed to those providing cover. For some animals, trees providing cover are assets, while for others they are a liability (Lima and Dill 1990; Miller 2002). Cover can both hide and impede vision as any infantry veteran who has experienced jungle combat knows. Ungulates such as zebra prefer open areas, not only for food but also for their evolved strategies for spotting predators. Their large group size is at the opposite pole of that needed for inconspicuousness. They rely more on speed, dilution and group defence and their stripes are thought to confuse predators' fixing their sights on any one individual. Their lesser reliance on relatedness can be observed by their apparent indifference to one of their group being taken before their eyes.

In the presence of large predators, being on the ground may be riskier than being up trees. Some species may be more at risk by day, others including ourselves by night. Some even have the capacity to switch these strategies when changing predation risks dictate this (Lima and Dill 1990). Further, for nocturnal animals it may be more dangerous to be out foraging during a full moon than a new moon.

Let us return one more time to surfing – catch the last wave of the day, though this is another dilemma as it can be risky. Aside from taking friends along as shark-bait, risks can be further reduced by avoiding surfing at dawn and dusk and avoiding river mouths, especially after heavy rain when nutrients are washed out into the sea, as shark feeding is increased at all these times. I have access to many local surf breaks, one of which is a rather sharky river mouth. The unusually aggressive bull shark frequents rivers. I ban myself from surfing the river mouth immediately after heavy rain, but in summer when the safer breaks are crowded with tourists, I do get tempted. With the increasing popularity of surfing and increasing coastal urbanization, some surfers are taking to surfing at night, preferably with the help of a full moon. Sharks are more active by night. This development exposes these surfers to sharks during periods of greater feeding activity. The shark that already has an overwhelming advantage has an even easier approach under the cover of dark. Forget it, I'm off to bed!

Primate foraging decision studies

Primates, because of their genetic relatedness to ourselves, are of greater interest in comparative studies than other animals. Unfortunately, there have been relatively few studies of primate foraging decisions under threat of predation. Studies of ring-tailed lemurs have produced data supporting the notion that predator sensitivity entails trade-offs between safety and foraging success in these primates (Sauther 2002; Miller 2002).

Adrian Treves (2002) has studied arboreal primates in this regard noting their three-dimensional capacity for cover and escape (up/down trees, sideways and forwards/backwards). Herd animals have a two-dimensional terrain (lacking the up/down). Predatory raptors (hawks, etc.) may have difficulty getting safely down trees close to the trunks to snatch monkeys. Leopards have difficulty getting up to them. Chimpanzees are heavy and have difficulty reaching prey monkeys on flimsy terminal branches. Treves (2002) predicted that wild red colobus monkeys (chimpanzees' favourite prey) would be more vigilant when foraging near the ground where they might be more at risk of a chimpanzee attack. Similarly, redtail monkeys, being prey for raptors, he predicted might be more vigilant when higher up in the canopy of trees. Third, he predicted that being a chimpanzee's delight, red colobus would be less vigilant when on terminal branches, while redtail monkeys being prey of raptors in such a position might be more vigilant.

Treves (2002) found that red colobus were more vigilant nearer the ground as predicted, but so were redtail monkeys, against his prediction. Both species were less vigilant near branch tips. He suggested the number of faulty predictions were more likely to be based on faulty assumptions about safety, as opposed to rejecting the otherwise well-supported findings from other studies that vigilance increases with risk of predation. Arboreal monkeys may vary their vigilance levels according to how readily they can see predators, not according to their own exposure. His study illustrates the early state of understanding primate defensive behaviour and the importance of avoiding premature assumptions, which will be particularly important when we explore these issues in early hominids.

Summary

Predation and foraging have been major pressures driving natural selection. Similar anti-predator 'decision-making' occurs in most species including insects, which lack cognitive capacity. Predator avoidance and anti-predator strategies have operated under different selection regimes with one reducing pressure on the other. Unsuccessful predation has been required for the evolution of anti-predator characteristics, because if predation were always successful there would be no prey to pass on the anti-predator genes. This selection issue reciprocally drives the selection of predator characteristics, but does so with less power. Anti-predator vigilance involves costs, particularly reduced time for feeding and reproductive activity. Costs can be reduced by group vigilance, but even this is associated with costs. Different species employ very different strategies, with group size ranging from huge to solitary individuals. The concept of predator-sensitive foraging can be approached by way of examining biological, social and environmental cost–benefit analyses involved in prey decision-making.

FAMILY FOIBLES AND EARLY HOMINIDS

Modern human behaviour is completely irrelevant to that of emergent hominids. Humans are the products of at least 2 million years of intense social evolution. Their mating and reproductive behaviours are saturated with religious, symbolic, and relational strictures. Almost no vertebrate species is less suited to the reconstruction of early hominid behaviour.

(Colin Lovejoy, 1982)

The pathway to humankind

Anthropologist Colin Lovejoy (1982) clearly overstated his case, but there is more than a grain of truth in his assertion. Indeed, we must be very cautious about extrapolating from the present to the past. The advent of civilization barely more than a blink of the eye ago has involved a particularly rapid phase of social development, heavily dependent on knowledge, communication and technological advances. Nevertheless, biosocial factors underlie much of our culture, especially when it comes to survival behaviours. For example, testosterone is a prerequisite for romance. Biology sets the agenda; culture elaborates it.

Lovejoy (1982) was concerned about the problems of using the present to reconstruct the past. My mission is the reverse. I will use the past era of early hominids to illuminate the probable innate defences of modern humans. Human personality evolutionary theory has been described as involving, first, the identification of adaptive problems confronted by ancestral human populations; second, the correlation of currently observable personality factors with the problems faced by ancestral populations; and third, the identification of inter-individual differences in their strategy deployment (Buss 1991). This book is about PTSD not personality, but there is a message here for the study of human defences. Simply put, how it was might be relevant to how it is.

Our distant ancestors (single celled creatures, early reptiles and early mammals) are useful for working out some of the ground rules, as we have seen. If we had a good understanding of our recent hominid ancestors we would be almost home and dry. However, there remains uncertainty as to even who should be included as our australopithecine and *Homo* ancestry, in what sequence and about their morphology. As for understanding their defensive and other behaviours, we have barely started. Hence, we still have to rely heavily on observations of other species, particularly primates and our great apes relatives. Our genetic similarity and physical structure suggest commonalities. These can be combined with findings from paleoanthropology and studies of hunter-gatherers.

I shall now review our lineage following our divergence from the common ancestor of humans, bonobos and chimpanzees. What follows is a simple summing-up that may not be accepted by many more expert than I in this area. It is the way in science that the current consensus is often a stereotypic portrait awaiting revision by the few experts at the cutting edge. Those at the cutting edge tend to disagree with each other and by the time their intellectual battles are resolved, new ones have arisen.

Hominids

Our hominid ancestors were ape-like but walked upright on two legs. The earliest hominids are referred to as australopithecines. Their era was from about 5 million to 1 million years ago (Wrangham and Peterson 1996). Australopithecines are sometimes referred to as 'woodland apes', as they were less confined to tropical rainforests than the other great apes. They lived in southern and central Africa. Although bipedal, they were closer to the other apes than humans, still possessing long arms for use in trees. They stood less than 5 foot (1.5 metres) tall. Their brain sizes were about one-third of ours, but similar to a chimpanzee's.

Australopithecus ramidus was one of the earliest australopithecines followed by *Australopithecus anamensis* and the better known *Australopithecus afarensis*, the first discovered of whom was nicknamed Lucy (named after the Beatles' song, 'Lucy in the Sky with Diamonds') (Fagan 1998). Lucy's brain size was still small, but her arms were only slightly longer than our own. Females may have been only 3 foot (1 metre) tall. There remains great controversy over this lineage and the diversification that followed, with the australopithecines going one way and the newcomer *Homo* another. *Australopithecus Africanus*, considered by some to be the first australopithecine, went off in one direction, being subsequently followed by the more robust skulled *Australopitheci Africanus*, *robustus* and *boisei* (Nategi 1995–1996a). Australopithecines coexisted with *Homo* for about 1 million years – a very long time compared with the 6000-year time span of written history.

Australopithecines developed into the *Homo* lineage, which commenced with *Homo habilis* ('habilis' means handyman) around 2.5 million years ago. *Homo habilis* was distinct from the australopithecines by having more human characteristics (Nategi 1995–1996b). Their brain was now over half the size of our own, but they still possessed long arms and greater sexual dimorphism. *Habilis* was still not much bigger than the australopithecines, but was more able to manipulate tools.

Like australopithecines, *habilis* ate mainly fruit and may not have been a regular hunter. *Habilis* probably scavenged from carnivores. Some 'prey' bones have been found to show stone tool cuts overlaying carnivore marks. The dangers of competing with carnivores may have been offset by better nutrition and so greater reproductive success (Fagan 1998). *Habilis* coexisted with a greater number of genera of large carnivores than exist nowadays in Africa (Treves, in preparation).

Homo erectus was the most important intermediary before *Homo sapiens*. *Homo erectus* arrived around 1.6 million years ago during the Great Ice Age of the Pleistocene period, at which time there were about five hominid species. *Erectus* stood around 6 foot

(1.8 metres) tall with a similar weight to ourselves. Improved ability to use technology allowed *erectus* to leave Africa for cooler parts of the world and still survive (Edlund 1995–1996). *Erectus* migrated northward along with other large animals, including predators. *Erectus* had a large brain and well-developed Broca's (speech) area. The enlarged brain may largely relate to increasingly complex human sociality (Dunbar 1996). *Erectus* butchered animals as large as elephants, but there is uncertainty as to whether they killed or merely scavenged them (Fagan 1998). By 1 million years ago *Erectus* was the sole surviving hominid. *Homo erectus* died out in all regions other than Africa where it developed into *archaic Homo sapiens* around 400,000 to 200,000 years ago (Fleming 1995–1996).

Archaic Homo sapiens neanderthalensis arrived around 130,000 years ago and was *sapiens'* European representative. The immensely strong neanderthals managed to adapt to the icy conditions and hunted large prey with strong spears. They persisted in Portugal up to about 28,000 years ago, coexisting with true *Homo sapiens*. Their bones have been found with large numbers of healed fractures, suggesting they cared for their injured (Geist 1978). The more slightly built Cro-Magnon, who was a later variant of *Homo sapiens*, used lighter throwing spears, suitable for smaller prey, mostly reindeer (Geist 1978). Cro-Magnon ventured into more varied conditions, including deserts where neanderthals could not operate successfully. Cro-Magnon had a higher forehead, suggesting expansion of the frontal lobes. Although neanderthals used tools, their tool development barely changed throughout their history (Gross 1992). The combination of a warmer climate, the greater numbers of Cro-Magnon and the latter's depletion of neanderthals' preferred prey through improved group hunting techniques, led to the extinction of neanderthals. Cro-Magnon coexisted with modern *Homo sapiens sapiens*, who were widely dispersed by at least 38,000 years ago (Gross 1992).

Following the Ice Age, the 'Neolithic' New Stone Age period started in South West Asia around 8000 BC, reaching parts of the Mediterranean coast as late as 4000 BC (Fagan 1998). Agriculture and village settlements developed. The arrival of agriculture brought spare time for activities other than food gathering such as the accumulation of wealth leading to greater stratification of society – the dawn of civilization.

In summary, while great uncertainty exists about the details of early hominids, we can safely conclude the following: hominids arrived about 200 million years after the advent of early mammals. About 5 million years ago australopithecines evolved from the common ancestor of the human, bonobo and chimpanzee lineages. The ape-like australopithecines evolved into the *Homo* species, which spread beyond Africa into more varied regions. *Homo* displayed massive increases in brain size and with this, greater complexity of social behaviours. On an evolutionary timescale *Homo sapiens sapiens* arrived virtually yesterday. Hence, our genetic make-up will overwhelmingly relate more to our earlier ancestors.

Primate and great ape extrapolations

Predation, though uncommon in present-day great apes, is still considered sufficient to exert selection pressure both by way of killing (removing genes) and by the fear of predation promoting effective anti-predator avoidance. Lions (Tsukahara 1993) and leopards (Boesch 1991) may kill chimpanzees. Orangutans of South East Asia are preyed upon by the clouded leopard and probably also bearded pigs, raptors and tigers (Setiawan et al. 1996). Even twenty-first century humans occasionally become victims to predators and have to modify their dwelling habits as a predator avoidance strategy.

While predation may have been the major threat to early primates, especially to the young, the old and the infirm, threats arose also from conspecifics, contributing to primate social systems. Female primates encountering unrelated males are at risk not only of coercive copulation, but also of having their dependants killed, and having their juveniles expelled from the group (Treves 1998). It is possible that the relatively monogamous 'permanent' pairing exemplified in the institution of marriage may have evolved as a strategy to reduce the great risk of killing of offspring by rival males (Ridley 1994). While gibbons seem to employ an essentially similar strategy to ourselves to prevent conspecific males killing their offspring, gorillas use the huge silverback 'minder'. Even now, human stepchildren are at far greater risk of being killed by their stepfathers, compared with the risk of children being killed by their biological fathers (Daly and Wilson 1988).

While predation pressure is likely to have been the dominant selection pressure before the arrival of the great apes, more recently apes have increasingly had to address the threat posed by conspecifics – both out-group and in-group ones. Recent defences will reflect conspecific pressures and involve more complex social behaviours, for example the social withdrawal (distinct from refuging) of PTSD. Let us now turn to great ape social groups. There are a few surprises to be found there.

Group size in great apes

The group size of a species will reflect defensive and other survival issues. We earlier established that increasing group size may reduce individual vigilance, freeing up more time for foraging (Lima 1995). However, vigilance and group size effects in primates are different from mammals in general. Primates evolved from predominantly non-gregarious ancestors (Treves 1998). In primates vigilance rarely reduces with increasing number of conspecific associates (Treves 2000). Unlike open plains animals, primates evolved in dense trop-ical rainforests. Increasing group size in primates carries the price of increased conspicuousness. Individual primate species have varying but small group sizes, which may also vary within a species according to food availability.

If inconspicuousness is a priority, how might primates reduce the costs of individual or small group vigilance? Vigilance for predators in primates is less influenced by numbers and more by their proxim-ity and social relatedness (Treves 2000). Primate vigilance strategies are strongly influenced by trust and reciprocity. Human war veterans tend to retain profound feelings of trust for their closer ex-comrades. Military training emphasizes the importance of protecting your mates.

Non-human primates direct a large proportion of their defensive vigilance at in-group conspecifics, as competition with associates is frequent and occasionally fatal (Treves 2000). Further, as might be expected, vigilance increases with increasing competition and subordinates direct more glances at associates than do dominants (Treves and Pizzagalli 2002). While intragroup vigilance may pose the most frequent need for vigilance, intergroup vigilance is associ-ated with greater danger per encounter. Predation and intragroup competition favour small group size, but this may not have been so for conspecific intergroup selection pressures.

The mainly fruit diet of early australopithecines would have exerted further selection pressure favouring small group size. As hominids left the rainforests for the savannahs, they developed dig-ging tools and the ability to tap the high energy resources of plant tubers. Being slow footed and not yet having invented weapons, australopithecines on the savannahs would still have had to rely on inconspicuousness.

Let us examine closely group sizes in the great apes (Figure 4.1). Orangutans arose from the first great apes to branch off from our common ancestor about 13 million years ago, followed by gorillas (9 million years ago), then hominids (5 million years ago), bonobos (2.5 million years ago), leaving the chimpanzee lineage as the most recent (Wrangham and Peterson 1996; Tanner 1987). As with hominids the chimpanzee lineage will have evolved since the first ancestral chimpanzees, although we do not know the details. Bonobos (pygmy chimpanzees) are very rare and were discovered only in 1928.

Orangutans are relatively solitary animals. Gorillas form groups typically consisting of a silverback male, three or four females and their offspring – around six to twelve individuals. The typical bonobo group size is eleven to fifteen individuals with a roughly equal male–female ratio. Chimpanzee party size ranges are remarkably small, usually being less than ten, often considerably so and rarely exceeding fifteen individuals, larger groups being constrained by both conspicuousness and food availability (Wrangham 1986; Wrangham and Peterson 1996). Chimpanzee parties often involve all males, with females frequently existing alone with their offspring and/or with a few other females (Susman 1987). Both chimpanzees and

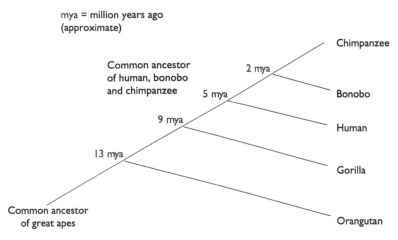

Figure 4.1 Great ape phylogeny
Source: adapted from Wrangham and Peterson 1996; Tanner 1987.

bonobos may aggregate into larger short-lived associations when food is plentiful.

Why should the group sizes of chimpanzees and remarkably similar bonobos differ? While defence was a major factor determining group size, so was the availability of food. It transpires that bonobos evolved in the rainforests south of the Zaire river after gorillas had left the region. Chimpanzees have had to compete with gorillas for plant food (Wrangham and Peterson 1996). Hence, 'gorilla food' is available to bonobos but harder to come by for chimpanzees. Not only does bonobo territory provide easier access to food, but also it promotes more cooperative and peaceful behaviour, in contrast to the more competitive chimpanzees.

While baboons are not great apes they merit a mention in the context of group size and social parallels with humans. They were studied as early as the 1800s as they shared some human environments. Research up to the early 1900s drew a number of erroneous conclusions about baboon and human similarities (Strum and Mitchell 1987). Nevertheless, baboons and early humans probably occupied similar ecological environments and there is no doubting that baboons are highly social. Baboons form larger groups than the non-human great apes, averaging between thirty and fifty individuals.

In baboons length of residency is a more important dimension than aggression-orientated dominance. Males new to the troop have been found to behave aggressively, presenting a show of dominance toward long-term residents, yet more peaceful long-term residents had greater success in accessing resources, including oestrus females. Non-aggressive social alternatives were used in both competition and defence (Strum and Mitchell 1987). It appears that being one of 'the club' counted for more than 'muscle'. Newcomers lack vital information and allies for social manoeuvring. Only 25 per cent of consort turnovers – winning another's female – were found to have resulted from aggression; most involved social skills with a female willing to respond to these. Further fighting was of no use unless a female allowed the male to copulate with her. As Strum and Mitchell (1987) stated, 'Manipulation and social intelligence clearly predate the human experiment.' The study did not determine whether early hominids behaved in this way. However, this possibility cannot be dismissed.

Before moving on from great ape group size, I will mention a simple experiment exploring human vigilance and group size, which came so close to delivering the golden egg. I hope that someone reading this may do the obvious follow-on. Wirtz and Wawra (1986) observed students at lunchtime in university cafeterias. Their key variables were: group size, sex and beginning and end of the periods during which students looked up from eating, apparently scanning the environment. Unfortunately they studied group sizes only up to five – i.e. the number of students typically eating at a table. They found vigilance was inversely proportional to group size (up to five). Also, in larger groups females reduced their rate of looking up from feeding more than males. This illustrates the potential experimental simplicity of exploring group size, vigilance and feeding in contemporary humans, with inferences about innate group sizes. Have you shared my experience of feeling self-conscious, not knowing quite where to look, while eating alone in public? What is the difference between self-consciousness and vigilance? Perhaps just a touch of egocentricity.

What Wirtz and Wawra (1986) did not demonstrate was at what group size might human vigilance while feeding reach a minimum, whether it then would rise (presumably it would) and the span of group sizes associated with less vigilant feeding. Had they done so, they might have discovered a major clue to the natural group size for humans, given our genes. However, this would still be context dependent, and our genes did not evolve for student cafeterias.

Finally on group size, let us note it was only recently in the Neolithic period from 12,000 years ago that aggression, including warfare, took off as a result of agriculture giving rise to the need to defend one's resources against raiders (Wrangham and Peterson 1996). Most of us do not have many more close friends than the group sizes of the great apes and baboons referred to above. The development of much larger human group sizes that comprise communities and nations nowadays may have been largely for the protection of massive resources, more a product of technology than evolution.

Beyond group size and social structure, research observations of primate anti-predator behaviour are limited. Avoidance of known dangerous areas and surveillance of surroundings are both universal among primates. The interval between predator detection and potential capture influences the anti-predator strategy selected. If the predator is detected at a distance, a number of defensive options may be employed. Quiet monitoring with or without alerting conspecifics may occur (Treves, in preparation). As with animals relying on large group defences, escape is the preferred option to confrontation.

However, unlike large group reliant animals, primates virtually always flee to refuges rather than trying to outrun their predators.

Less commonly, primates may stand their ground in the face of predators, in which case mobbing might be employed. This involves noisy warnings to deter approach by the predator. This defence involves not only intimidation, but also distraction and confusion. Chimpanzees may occasionally kill leopards. Nevertheless, it is unlikely that early hominids would have been capable of reliably killing larger prey before the advent of sophisticated weaponry. Furthermore, the effectiveness of counterattack with weapons is reduced if caught by surprise (Treves, in preparation).

Primate research limitations

Great ape social structures and defence

Before examining defences employed by early hominids I will review those of non-human great apes. Both out-group and in-group conspecific threats need to be considered. Contemporary non-human great apes, our closest living relatives, could hardly be a more different bunch.

Orangutans are the least social of the great apes. Mother–infant or juveniles are the only stable social units (Wrangham and Peterson 1996). Males lead solitary existences. Orangutan females are regularly raped, but the lack of male-initiated infanticide is one of their redeeming features. In all these respects, their psychology is very different from our own.

Gorillas are much more social, but have social units quite unlike our own. They involve the hugely dimorphic silverback males who protect their three or four females and juveniles, leading an existence second only for affection and peacefulness to the bonobo (Wrangham and Peterson 1996). The silverback's idea of aggression directed at approaching male strangers is usually only a grand display of bravado – pure bluff. However, when a male outsider ousts a silverback – nobody dominates forever – the new male frequently kills the females' offspring, as they do not carry his genes and he will inherit many domestic duties. Female gorillas are pragmatic; they accept the loss of their infants and get on with making new ones with their new protector. Otherwise, their reproductive future would be bleak and their genes disadvantaged.

Bonobos are the most peaceful of the apes and have two

outstanding social characteristics. First, they engage in high frequency hetero- and homo-sexual activity with adults and youngsters. Second, females cooperate effectively with other females, in contrast to males that rarely cooperate (except sexually) with other males (Wrangham and Peterson 1996). Both female cooperation and the male lack of this contribute to the successful limiting of male aggression despite their greater size and strength. The male bonobo is tamed by his Venus in their garden of promiscuity.

Chimpanzees are remarkably similar-looking to the bonobo though larger. Male chimpanzees regularly batter females into submission and rape is common. Small groups of a few males dominate their social systems. Females generally prefer to forage individually (Wrangham 1979). Females protect their offspring by copulating with all the neighbouring males, thereby making their infants potential offspring of any of the males. Accordingly the males are less likely to kill the juveniles, as they might be their own (Wrangham and Peterson 1996). Chimpanzees may use weapons against large prey such as leopards, which they may club with branches (Boesch 1991).

Anthropologist Richard Wrangham described a chimpanzee troop undergoing fission (dividing into two subgroups) (Wrangham 1999a; Wrangham and Peterson 1996). Subsequently one subgroup repeatedly raided the other over four years. Progressively the raiders eliminated the other subgroup's males amidst much excitement. They did not do this to gain access to females for breeding, as they then proceeded to kill all the females until the other subgroup was completely eliminated. An implication of these observations is that the ancestral apes that gave rise to humans and chimpanzees may have evolved genes for coalitionary killing (Wrangham 1999a). If agriculture has been a key factor in the escalation of collective human warfare, let us hope chimpanzees never discover the plough.

This rather stereotypic description of our great ape relatives emphasizes the diversity in behaviours and social structures that may emerge despite genetic similarity. Accordingly, extrapolations to human social structures must be approached cautiously.

Primate inferences for hominids

With this caution in mind, what might we safely surmise from primate research with respect to our probable genetic defensive make-up? First, hominids would have been the exception among the great apes if they were to derive safety from large group formation.

The largest group size of other apes is in the highly social bonobo, which typically forms groups of around a dozen individuals. The larger brain of *Homo sapiens* also suggests more complex capacity for socialization and larger group size. Allowing for this and an adjustment taking into account the social commonalities of *Homo* and baboons, perhaps the early *Homo* group size might have been in the region of those of bonobos to baboons – say ten to thirty individuals or more conservatively, five to fifty (five being a typical chimpanzee small group size and fifty being a large baboon group size). This is far smaller than the quaintest village communities of the present day. Second, the evidence clearly points to hominids being vulnerable to not only predation but also conspecific intergroup and intragroup killing of adults and unrelated offspring. Infanticide by males would have required some sort of social defence strategy by mothers.

Predation and intragroup competition would favour small group sizes. Larger groups may have defended themselves better against intergroup conspecific raids, but their group size would have been limited by the availability of food. Third, prior to weapon making, hominids would have had difficulty defending themselves at close quarters against carnivores. They may have utilized mobbing as a defence, but generally only when close to a last resort. If predators were detected by early hominids, they would have preferred flight and combined this with the use of refuges such as trees. Mostly they would have pursued inconspicuousness to avoid detection by predators.

Paleoanthropology

Paleoanthropology uses data from traces of hominids and their environmental settings to reconstruct hominid behaviour and ecology (Potts 1987). Three types of evidence are used: hominid fossils, paleoenvironmental data and archaeological data. Fossils may provide, for example, reliable information on body size, sexual dimorphism, locomotion, hand function and diet. Paleoenvironmental evidence gives rise to four major areas of research. Sedimentary studies may elucidate aspects of the environment such as lakes, lake margins, delta and riverine zones; geochemical studies provide evidence of climatic conditions; plant fossils suggest the floral environment; and faunal remains are another source of information (Potts 1987). Archaeological evidence of hominid behaviour and ecology is limited, but includes stone tools, techniques of their manufacture, and functions of some artefacts. Digging sticks, for example, would have greatly increased their food supply.

Our present-day world is a utopia. Early hominids were prey to false sabre tooth cats and other large predators. Most humans in the developed nations live in environments almost free from predators, with substantially reduced conspecific violence (war excepted), premature death and other traumas compared with our hominid ancestors.

The earliest hominids would have lived in tropical forests and occasionally copulated with ancestral apes. Their ability to stand carried a number of advantages as well as costs. With their upright stance and free arms, hominids learnt to dig for carbohydrate-rich tubers, resources that were untouched by other foragers. They could even carry them home. This led to their range extending beyond the rainforests into lowland woodland, into the savannah and eventually out of Africa (Wrangham and Peterson 1996).

Hominids as scavengers and prey

Australopithecines were commonly prey for leopards. Several African cave sites dated between 1 million and 3 million years ago have revealed fossilized remains of large carnivores along with those of 140 australopithecines and 324 baboons (Treves, in preparation). Remains of the larger primates have shown characteristic patterns of damage by large cats and hyenas. *Dinofelis*, the false sabre tooth cat, was about the size of a small lion and had a tooth shape intermediate between modern cats and the true sabre tooths. *Dinofelis* may have specialized in preying on australopithecines and baboons. Hominids not only were hunted but also encountered predators during their scavenging activities. Although the extent to which hominids were preyed upon is unclear, there is evidence that remains of hominids were taken back to the dens of carnivores.

Early carnivores would have little reason to fear early hominids. There is no evidence of the use of stone tools before 2.5 million years ago or of the controlled use of fire before 2 million years ago (Treves, in preparation). Even with the advent of these new defences, they would have been of modest value against the surprise attacks of large predators.

Early hominids would most probably have been wary of caves and other locations where large predators might be lurking. Hominids in open country would have been constrained by lack of refuges (Treves 2000, 2002). In woodlands, refuges were plentiful but obstructed vigilance would have been a concern. Treves (in preparation) suggests:

> Modern humans may retain traces of some of the anti-predator adaptations of our ancestors. In particular, predictable behavioural responses and aversion to areas with dense vegetation or areas without suitable refuge (e.g., wide, open areas) should be deeply embedded in human cognitive and perceptual abilities.

It may be that 'park-like' settings with a combination of trees for hiding, but openness for predator and intergroup conspecific detection, combined with lakes or rivers may have been the preferred hominid environment.

Plio-Pleistocene hominids ate a higher quality diet than contemporary baboons and given the larger average mass of hominids, Treves (in preparation) suggests foraging group sizes exceeding twenty individuals would have been unlikely. He proposes that hominids would have adopted a relatively calm cohesive social organization maintaining vigilance, cooperating and reducing conspicuousness.

Potts (1987) reviewed findings from the archaeological site of Bed I Olduvai Gorge in Tanzania. Stone tools, other artefacts and broken animal bones from various species traditionally had been interpreted as suggesting a home base for food sharing and social activity of hominids. However, it was evident that animal bones were brought to the site over several years, much longer than that over which modern tropical hunter-gatherers would occupy their campsites. Second, examination of bones revealed damage inflicted by carnivore teeth as well as hominid stone tools over the entire period of site use. The co-occurrence of hominids and carnivores would have been incompatible with safety. Also the bones from Olduvai were not as intensively modified as at modern campsites. Potts (1987) suggested the stone tools and bones at such sites represent 'stone caches' where tools could be located and prey could be quickly processed – an early form of meatworks. Large carnivores attracted to such sites by the scents would compete for the food resources.

Another way to explore the likely behaviour of our ancestors is to examine behaviour in contemporary humans as far from the effects of civilization as possible. Treves (1998) studied competition between modern humans and carnivores in Uganda. He tapped the Ugandan Game Department Archives (UGDA), which recorded human–wildlife conflict from 1923 to 1994 to protect both wildlife and humans from each other. He found nine reports of humans scavenging from lion and leopard kills. Three records made anecdotal references to human scavenging of carnivore prey being common. This further suggests that scavenging from predators may have been a strategy widely employed by ancestral hominids.

Hunter-gatherers

Contemporary study of the few remaining hunter-gatherers of the new world emphasizes the likely selection pressure arising from human conspecifics in the later stages of our evolution. The Ache, natives of Paraguay, until recently were full-time nomadic foragers. The median size of their bands was forty-eight, only slightly larger than the size suggested for early hominids. Recent life for the Ache has involved about 20 per cent of their children dying before the age of 1 year and about 40 per cent dying by the age of 15. Homicide has accounted for 31 per cent of Ache child mortality. Comparable homicide data are available for two other hunter-gatherer groups (Hill and Hurtado 1989): 14 per cent of Hiwi but only 4 per cent of !Kung San (Kalahari Bushmen) childhood deaths are by homicide. Among Ache adults, warfare and accidents accounted for 73 per cent of total mortality, compared with 39 per cent of Hiwi and only 11 per cent of !Kung San. These findings suggest high levels of human conspecific-induced mortality. A study of the !Kung San, now known as the Ju/hoansi, found that they suffered PTSD but had fewer avoidance symptoms than found in modern cultures (McCall and Resick 2003).

Human defensive evolution since the advent of hominids has occurred in three phases: first, small groups defending against predators; second, similar but also hunting large game; and third, defending against other human groups giving rise to warfare (Alexander 1979). Analysis of fifty hunter-gatherer societies revealed that 64 per cent engaged in warfare at least once every two years (Ember 1978). Among thirteen human raiding cultures, the median percentage of male deaths caused by conspecific violence was found to be 20–30 per cent, similar to an estimate for chimpanzees (Wrangham 1999b). The territoriality and resource acquisitioning associated with agriculture have driven the development of warfare. It is possible that agriculture may not have given rise to collective violence per se, but merely to collective violence on a more massive scale.

While predation pressure dominated early ancestral defence selection, conspecific pressure seems most relevant to very recent developments. These influences might be expected to have left anatomical imprints in MacLean's triune brain.

Summary

Early hominid defence can be approached via three main avenues: primatology, paleoanthropology and studies of contemporary hunter-gatherers. Despite genetic similarities the social structures of the different great apes are diverse. Nevertheless, all great apes have relied on inconspicuousness. This requires small group sizes, preferably combined with trustworthy comrades, such as kin. The great ape defences and probable hominid diet suggest the typical early hominid group size would have probably been only a few dozen individuals. Paleoanthropology suggests that the earliest hominids were more likely to have been the prey of larger carnivores than the reverse. They were also scavengers competing with carnivores. More recently, the advent of weapons and fire would have afforded better defence against large carnivores, but conspecifics would have been a major cause of mortality and selection pressure.

Chapter 5

Defence in overdrive
Evolution, PTSD and parsimony

> He that will not apply new remedies must expect new evils, for time
> is the greatest innovator.
>
> Francis Bacon, 1561–1626

Stearns and Hoekstra (2000) commented, 'When experiments are possible, they yield more reliable insights than comparisons, but a well controlled comparison is more informative than a nonexistent experiment.' The present comparisons of PTSD symptoms with animal defences suggest an overall theory from which more specific ideas and hypotheses emerge. The latter are testable and will ultimately determine the value of the underlying theory.

Thus far, I have described PTSD, some conventional theories of its causes that are mostly proximate in orientation, reviewed basic evolutionary theory and presented some animal research on defensive reactions. From here on I will describe the evolutionary theory of PTSD and its components with the above in mind.

An evolutionary theory of PTSD

At a symptom level the basic evolutionary theory I am proposing suggests that the re-experiencing phenomena of PTSD represent higher order memory and learning experiences. These experiences are associated with hypervigilance (watchfulness) and avoidance behaviours. Simply put, if ancestral individuals have had seriously threatening experiences, their long-term survival might be promoted if their lessons were not forgotten (re-experiencing symptoms); if they remained for an extended period on high alert (overarousal symptoms); if they avoided high-risk locations and activities (avoidance behaviours); and were quick to use other defences as determined by contextual demands.

Intrusive recollections have been found to intensify over time in those who develop PTSD (Yehuda et al. 1998). However, over the duration of PTSD, re-experiencing phenomena fade more quickly than avoidance behaviours and overarousal symptoms. This might be explained by the suggestion that if memory has succeeded in producing a more cautious orientation to life, the ongoing re-experiencing 'lessons' need not be so harsh or repeated.

Vigilance, avoidance and flight have obvious potential survival value, even if overgeneralized – it is better to be safe than sorry. It seems indisputable that 'avoidance behaviours' reflect avoidance and other defensive phenomena.

PTSD symptom criteria revisited

Having briefly described the skeleton of the theory, I will now relate it to the clinical phenomena according to the DSM-IV criteria (APA 1994). The DSM-IV criteria are not comprehensive. There are other symptoms that occur that are not officially listed, some of which may be more important than is currently recognized. The criteria currently used are considered important and sufficient for making the diagnosis. They are not cast in stone; they have already changed in successive DSM revisions.

Let us now examine them in their current form from the perspective of their likely defensive origins and functions in evolutionary history. In Chapter 2, I presented the five DSM-IV re-experiencing phenomena, codes B1 to B5. Intrusive recollections (code B1) appear akin to exaggerated memory. They intrude into everyday situations and refuse to go away. Severe intrusive recollections, for example of a serious car accident, may make conversation difficult. By keeping the trauma at the forefront of the mind, such recollections result in more cautious driving or avoidance of it altogether.

Nightmares (B2) also appear to have a clear memory function; many sufferers would dearly love to be able to forget them. But might they not also be overarousal symptoms? Patients commonly report waking up from nightmares so drenched in sweat that they feel inclined to change the sheets. I previously suggested that individual defensive phenomena might serve more than one function. Hence, it would not be surprising if specific symptoms similarly crossed the DSM categories. The hippocampus is responsible for selecting important memories such as those relating to survival, especially the contextual elements of these, and relaying them to the cortex for long-term storage (Davis and Whalen 2001). However, this process is lengthy, taking around two years to be complete, with multiple replays from the hippocampus to the cortex. Furthermore, it seems that much of this occurs during sleep. Nightmares consolidate this transfer of information ensuring it will not be forgotten in the long term (Carter 1998).

Acting or feeling as though the traumatic event was recurring (B3) seems to have a strong associative element, but again may also involve an element of overarousal. Consider a bank teller with PTSD who looks up and freezes as she sees a young man with a hooded jacket vaguely resembling the man who held her up previously.

Intense psychological distress in response to 'cues that symbolize or resemble an aspect of the traumatic event' (B4) has a clear memory element, as does physiological reactivity on exposure to reminders (B5). Yet again, it can be argued that they also have an overarousal component. They also strongly overlap with avoidance behaviours. One probing question commonly employed with these two symptoms is, 'Does television coverage of violence or other themes relevant to your trauma cause you undue distress?' Patients commonly respond that they do not watch television news or other programmes featuring violence and thereby avoid this scenario.

In the avoidance behaviours, criterion C1 is avoiding thoughts, feelings or conversations associated with the trauma. It is a vital component of Horowitz's (1986) notion of oscillation – as the traumatic recollections enter the individual's mind he/she strives to get rid of them. It probably represents psychological flight as well as avoidance. Generally to 'avoid' thinking about something, you have to have first considered it, before choosing to flee from and thereafter avoid it. Re-experiencing symptoms and the high alert of overarousal/hypervigilance phenomena keep psychological avoidance/flight high on the individual's agenda.

Efforts to avoid activities, places or people that arouse recollections of the trauma (C2) are quite clearly the first rule of defence: don't expose yourself to danger, then you won't have to flee, let alone fight. Although the bases of most defensive responses may have been laid down in the reptilian era, the limited aerobic capacity of reptiles and their predecessors suggest that some aspects of the flight/fight responses would have developed in the mammalian eras (MacLean 1949). The avoidance criteria are more about avoidance than flight.

A lizard may hide motionless in a crack in a rock for much of the day, emerging for the essentials of energy acquisition and reproduction at low-risk times. Hence, predator avoidance reduces the necessity for flight, which requires greater aerobic capacity.

Avoidance and flight are different but inextricably linked. The turtle illustrates the overlap between avoidance and flight most graphically. Its active though energy-undemanding withdrawal into its shell is a highly effective 'flight', but its avoidance by way of not coming out till danger has passed is undeniable.

It is commonplace to set patients exposure therapy tasks, such as visiting a supermarket, only for them to fail to get into their car to go to the supermarket, or to get there and promptly flee. The two phenomena avoidance and flight tend to be seen by clinicians as one and the same. This is incorrect as different gene-neural mechanisms are involved (Brodie et al. 1991). I will return to this later.

Inability to recall an important aspect of the trauma (C3) is a form of avoidance involving dissociation and is particularly common in those abused as children (van der Kolk 1996b). Chapters 8 and 9 have much to add in this regard.

Avoidance criteria C4 to C6 are problematic, all reflecting the same problem. They are, to remind you: markedly diminished interest or participation in significant activities (C4); feelings of detachment or estrangement from others (C5); restricted range of affect (e.g. unable to have loving feelings) (C6). All three include emotional numbing as well as social withdrawal/flight elements. Female victims of assault not only are at greater risk of developing PTSD, but also experience more numbing symptoms than male victims (Breslau et al. 1999). Foa et al. (1992) have suggested separating these numbing symptoms from avoidance behaviours and evolutionary reasoning supports this. For numbing to be a useful defence some level of engagement with the threat would be necessary. Avoiding a predator does not require distraction from pain – flight and fight do.

The common reptilian response of refuging – retreating into an inaccessible crevice or other haven – may have been the prototype for present-day housebound states associated with PTSD. Although the DSM-IV caters for social withdrawal, it does not appear to recognize the importance of refuging – i.e. withdrawal to a sanctuary. It also does not recognize the independence of avoidance, flight and numbing, which are likely to be mediated by different gene-neural mechanisms yet may all superficially appear to belong in category C5. We saw earlier that predator avoidance and anti-predation strategies are under different selection regimes with the development of one easing the pressure on the other (Brodie et al. 1991).

Avoidance criterion C7, a sense of a foreshortened future (e.g., does not expect to have a career, marriage, children, or a normal lifespan) has a submissive yielding quality – subordinates communicating to more dominant conspecifics. However, it is a particularly blurred criterion as it has the pessimistic, even suicidal overtones that overlap too much with depression to be really useful. Evolutionary theory suggests that losses giving rise to depression differ in mechanisms from the defence-related traumas giving rise to PTSD. Their gene-neural bases are quite distinct (Panksepp 1998).

The overarousal category conceptualization is the one of the three which appears most confused. There are numerous types of arousal for example, sexual, optimistic excitement (elation), pessimistic excitement (dread), fear and so on. PTSD overarousal presumably reflects the fear variety. In which case might the concept of hypervigilance be a more appropriate conceptual basis than overarousal symptoms? The overarousal DSM-IV criteria: difficulty falling or staying asleep (D1), hypervigilance (D4) and exaggerated startle response (D5) suggest vigilance phenomena – vigilance being a forerunner to decisive defensive action. The use of the term 'hypervigilance' for category D4 is most unfortunate. In clinical practice I find D4 to be one of the most useful categories, if approached as a tendency to *feel wary in a variety of situations.* Hypervigilance ethologically implies watchfulness. This concept may be more useful than, but does not negate, the physiological notion of overarousal.

In depression people may lie awake worrying about their losses or problems, but it is fear that keeps those with PTSD awake – the fear that something bad is about to happen. It almost seems vindicated when a bump in the night justifies the individual getting up to investigate. This is quite different from the sleep problems associated with depression. The DSM wording should better reflect this to reduce the potential for diagnostic confusion from this otherwise useful criterion.

Startle reactions are the fastest defensive response of all, a mixture of vigilance, aggression and confusion (in the attacker) generating elements that buy fractions of, or a few seconds of, time before some more definitive action may be needed. The reflexive nature of an exaggerated startle response suggests a reptilian origin. Sure enough from the perspective of functional neuroanatomy, mammalian startle reactions appear to arise from a relatively simple neuronal circuit located in the lower (reptilian) brainstem (Koch 1999).

Criteria D2 and D3 are particularly out of place from an evolutionary perspective. Irritability and outbursts of anger (D2) clearly reflect aggressive defence. As one of the four fundamental mammalian defences I will give it in-depth coverage in Chapter 7, so I will not elaborate at this stage other than to note that from an evolutionary perspective, this key defence sits in stark isolation within a group of mostly hypervigilance phenomena.

As for the remaining criterion, difficulty concentrating (D3), this is even more unfortunate. While it could be driven by overarousal or hypervigilance phenomena, it could also be driven by numbing, as in being emotionally shut down – the inverse of overarousal. Even from the phenomenological as opposed to evolutionary perspective, this scenario would appear unsupportable. This problem could be simply solved by better wording – e.g. difficulty concentrating because of overarousal. This assumes that we have successfully replaced the 'overarousal' (D1–D5) category label with 'hypervigilance'.

The evolutionary perspective sheds new light on these diagnostic criteria, suggesting potential modifications. It is important to recognize that criteria do not need to represent all symptoms; they should be the minimum that produce valid and reliable results. If a single symptom or category of symptoms were both universal and diagnostic of PTSD, one would suffice for diagnostic purposes – but not for understanding the problem. Variable interpretations of PTSD boundaries by experts at times have attracted scathing criticisms in the law courts. Boundaries are particularly open to interpretation with regards to depression and specific phobias.

The current DSM-IV scheme has memory, vigilance and avoidance categories. Might more than one of the six broad mammalian behavioural defences warrant category status? To recap, these are avoidance, withdrawal or flight, aggressive defence, appeasement and the two immobilities. Flight as we have seen has been confused with avoidance. Depressed individuals may avoid going to shopping centres, but they generally do not flee from them in fear. Specific phobics may do so if shopping centres are part of their phobias, but not otherwise. People with specific phobias do not tend to be unusually irritable (aggressive defence), but depressives commonly are. Appeasement is specific to complex PTSD. The two immobilities are too fleeting for independent diagnostic category status.

Where does this leave us? First, I suggest that complex PTSD warrants a specific diagnostic status as a subtype and one with specific representation of appeasement in a separate symptom category. The criteria for ordinary PTSD might be improved by tightening the avoidance category to separate avoidance from flight (and numbing). Flight is probably as universal in PTSD as avoidance. Some sufferers even develop new avoidance behaviours because of their traumatic humiliation of, for example, having fled from a supermarket without their groceries. Epidemiological studies have not addressed this, as flight has been incorrectly subsumed under avoidance. Hence, some flight criteria might warrant a separate category. This would go some way to eliminating confusion with depression. Generalized irritability/explosivity is common in PTSD. Listing it in a separate category might reduce confusion with specific phobias. However, as it is not universal it could not stand alone. Perhaps it might be placed in a miscellaneous category embracing not only aggressive defence, but also the transient immobilities and numbing (a physiological defence already recognized as out of place in the avoidance category: Foa et al. 1992).

Adaptive or maladaptive: the relevance of subthreshold states

If PTSD is a disorder of defence, this suggests neurologically either it must use existing brain wiring to produce the manifestations of the disorder, or it must utilize circuitry that is not normally employed in defensive behaviours, but which can mimic defensive circuitry. The latter seems unlikely. A more parsimonious explanation is that it uses what is already there – the existing circuitry of defence mechanisms, which will have many similarities across species. This suggests that evolution will yield many neuroscientific clues about PTSD's fundamental wiring and activation. Current 'pathology'-based theories suggesting unpredictable aberrations might be replaced with a more predictable evolutionary understanding of PTSD that may integrate neuroanatomy, neurochemistry, memory, information processing, learning, behavioural and other conceptualizations.

One of the key questions about PTSD from an evolutionary perspective is whether it is adaptive, maladaptive or just an aberration with little or no evolutionary basis. If it is an aberration it is unlikely to exist widely in the animal kingdom. Veterinary medicine is starting to suggest it exists in domestic animals (Dodman and Shuster

1998), but at this stage the *research evidence* is lacking. However, this is so because of failure to consider this possibility, as opposed to negative evidence. If PTSD is found to be widely distributed across species, this still would not unequivocally determine whether PTSD has been adaptive over evolutionary time, but it would suggest this – maladaptive traits tend to die out over long time periods. Its persistence in the more ancient species would further support adaptiveness.

Adaptation is a state that evolved because it improved reproductive performance, to which survival contributes (Stearns and Hoekstra 2000). What is adaptive in an evolutionary sense may be disabling at an individual level. I have lost count of the numbers of soldiers, police and security officers I have seen who developed severe PTSD in response to occupational traumas and as a result have become unable to continue their dangerous careers. They have had to leave these lifestyles, with obvious implications from an evolutionary perspective. However, surely our ancestral environments were even more dangerous and so might be expected to be even more disabling? Two points are relevant here. First, remember the research on predictability reducing anxiety in hazardous environments and my suggestion that motor racers generally quickly recover psychologically from horrific accidents, in large part because of expectations. Second, a small dose of PTSD with hypervigilance, avoidance of hazards, aggression, etc. may have promoted survival in such environments. Occasionally even a large dose in the present time may be adaptive, as we shall later see.

Evolutionary adaptive theory includes maladaptations. Accordingly, even if PTSD is detrimental to the transmission of genes to further generations, and perhaps peculiar to humans, evolutionary theory may still point the way. Maladaptation may result when genes flow to a niche for which they did not evolve (Stearns and Hoekstra 2000). Maladaptations are adaptations for a different time or place. An aggressive temperament, for example, may be an asset in wartime but not during peace when sensitivity may be preferred. While at times PTSD may still be adaptive, much of the time it will be maladaptive. Our dated genes for defence may not suit the needs of our wonderful experiment called civilization.

The irritability and anxiety associated with PTSD does not favour mate attraction. Furthermore, sexual dysfunction is commonly associated with PTSD. Both factors might contribute to lower reproductive success rates. At first glance these appear to be phenomena that would be selected against. However, the cost of lost insemination opportunities might be offset by the greater family defensive orientation in contexts demanding this. In hostile environments reproductive success may be better promoted by protecting what you have, as opposed to producing other vulnerable beings that may jeopardize those already there. The same genetic make-up may result in both adaptation and maladaptation depending on the context.

A crucial element of the question of whether PTSD might be adaptive or maladaptive is the issue of subclinical, or more accurately, sub-diagnostic threshold PTSD. Clinical as opposed to community-based samples often create categorical illusions. Down's syndrome is a categorical disorder. People do not have a little bit of it; they have it or they do not. In contrast depression, anxiety and many other psychiatric disorders are more likely to exist on a continuous spectrum with normality – they are dimensional. A central issue is whether psychiatric disorders are separated from one another, and from normality, by zones of rarity (Kendell and Jablensky 2003).

Let us consider PTSD research from the perspective of whether PTSD symptomatology is associated with discrete cut-offs from normality.

One study found that as many as 95 per cent of rape victims showed PTSD symptoms within one to two weeks of the crime (Foa 1997). Clearly this reaction was the norm. This rate declined to 60 per cent at four weeks and 51 per cent at twelve weeks. Similarly, a study of the Oklahoma City bombing in 1995, which had a death toll of 167, found that the full PTSD criteria were met by one-third of survivors, but some PTSD symptoms were nearly universal – experiencing some PTSD symptoms was the rule (North et al. 1999). Ruscio et al. (2002), using three taxometric statistical procedures on a large sample of veterans exposed to extreme combat stress, found results supported PTSD being dimensional with PTSD representing one extreme. The police research cited in Chapter 3 also suggests that trauma symptoms may be dimensional.

The question I posed was whether PTSD was adaptive, maladaptive or just an aberration? The above considerations suggest the question should be reframed. Has PTSD been adaptive *and* maladaptive, *or* just an aberration? I favour the former, which gives rise to the question of under which circumstances is PTSD adaptive and under which is it maladaptive? The answer depends on the contexts, which we will see warrant far closer consideration than is usual in PTSD research.

Conclusions

The evolutionary theory views re-experiencing symptoms as the mechanism by which learning, memory and prioritization of defence memories have occurred, following seriously threatening exposure to dangers. Avoidance behaviours reflect avoidance, flight and numbing phenomena. The overarousal category of symptoms might be better conceptualized as hypervigilance phenomena, encompassing both ethological and physiological vigilance. DSM-IV criteria might be improved by some consideration of mammalian defences.

PTSD is a disorder of defence that is likely to use existing brain neurocircuitry-controlling defensive functions. PTSD may well exist in many species, in which case much might be learnt by studying animals, preferably in their natural environments for which their defences evolved. PTSD may well have been adaptive over evolutionary time, but may be adaptive in some and maladaptive in other past and present contexts. If PTSD is viewed as existing on a continuum with normality it is likely that much of the adaptiveness of the state derives from subthreshold levels of severity.

Chapter 6

Perspectives and possibilities

Vigilance, avoidance and attentive immobility

It is easy to be brave from a safe distance.
Aesop, 620–560 BC

A small band of vigilant australopithecines wait downwind from a cave used by a false sabre tooth cat that made a large kill the day before. It cannot have consumed such a quantity of food. They do not have spears, for these have yet to be invented. Even though there are a dozen of them, they must avoid contact with this predator, as they would be defenceless if confronted by it. They are hungry and take calculated risks. Having observed the cave from their hiding place, they see a cat emerge. When it has travelled a safe distance, they pursue their opportunity for a large piece of its catch. As they approach the entrance to the cave, they hear a noise from within and, as one, freeze . . .

Vigilance

Having proposed an evolutionary basis for PTSD and examined it from a clinical perspective let us now revisit the mammalian defences and see what flows from these considerations. For many millions of years defence has been fundamental for survival. Despite inter-species diversity of defences, there is a great deal of uniformity when it comes to overall behavioural strategies. In mammals defensive behavioural strategies can be conceptualized as sixfold and loosely in the following sequence: avoidance, followed by flight and then aggressive defence, with attentive immobility diffusely crossing boundaries, appeasement, and finally tonic immobility. I further suggest that vigilance and risk assessment are precursors to all these defences. The next four chapters will proceed on this basis.

The selection of defences against predators, conspecifics or environmental threats, requires threat detection, assessment of context and defence strategy selection. In keeping with 'prey decision-making' such analyses may occur anywhere along the spectrum from reflex to cognitive levels. These levels of analyses may occur simultaneously and reach different conclusions. Older brain structures may signal threat and activate behaviours accordingly, while cognitions signal no threat, causing confusion, which happens to be one of the most distressing aspects of PTSD.

While neuroscientists and clinicians usually define vigilance in terms of a brain state of receptivity to external stimuli directly associated with alertness, ethologists may define vigilance as looking up from foraging or simply as a visual search of the environment beyond the immediate vicinity (Treves and Pizzagalli 2002). Although vigilance suggests 'watchfulness' as in sight, I will take it to include all the special senses. In jungle warfare, sound may be the dominant vigilant sense aided even by smell. There are many accounts from Vietnam of troops who failed to recognize that the enemy might be able to smell them, their cigarette smoke, and their more pungent faeces associated with their richer western diet of meat.

Avoidance implies watchfulness. Before the more active defences, flight or fight, can be employed, detection must occur. Vigilance will be a precondition to selecting all defensive responses. Hence, neurodevelopmentally one might expect it to be represented in the older reptilian brain areas. Sure enough the site in the brain with a major responsibility for arousal, attention and their vigilant behavioural manifestations is the reticular activating system located in the midbrain in the upper reaches of the brainstem.

Ethologically, hypervigilance or 'overarousal' might be more accurately termed 'higher arousal' without the value judgement. When this is borne in mind the relevance of context becomes much more pertinent. I will regard vigilance as a behavioural state involving alertness and scanning for dangers. While an ethological perspective of vigilance may be an improvement on the purely physiological conceptualization of arousal, it can be improved still further. Neither watchfulness nor heightened arousal themselves provide useful behavioural functions in isolation. Risk assessment is the key function of vigilance (Blanchard et al. 1991). It is particularly relevant to ambiguous threats and thereby to PTSD. Readiness for a rapid and definitive defensive response is the key function of physiological arousal that operates in conjunction with hypervigilance.

The evolutionary theory suggests that the first step in the process of developing PTSD is registering and remembering the trauma, through re-experiencing symptoms; the second step is heightened vigilance; and the third step is the use of avoidance and other defences. While almost all survivors of the 1995 Oklahoma City bombing experienced some PTSD symptoms, re-experiencing and overarousal symptoms were more prevalent than avoidance behaviours, which were more associated with full-blown PTSD, found in only one-third of survivors (North et al. 1999). This and other studies (Kulka et al. 1990; Galea et al. 2002b) point to subclinical levels of PTSD being common.

Lesser reactions, experienced by the majority of such trauma survivors, were effectively to readily recall (re-experience) the tragic events and be highly vigilant for further dangers. In the 2003 terrorist alert, Australian television relayed political messages to viewers consisting essentially of: 'Remember we are living in unusually dangerous times . . . be vigilant . . . but go about your normal lives and don't avoid things unnecessarily.' The adaptiveness of this message is self-evident.

Predator-sensitive foraging and PTSD: fertile pasture or blind alley?

Vigilance, often alternating with feeding activity, is common in virtually all higher animals (Blanchard et al. 1991). It is intuitive that in more dangerous circumstances organisms should be more vigilant. But, it may be asked, why not be more vigilant all the time? If prey are overly cautious they may miss valuable feeding or mating opportunities, while if they are insufficiently so the consequences may fatal. An 'apprehension continuum' is dependent on a cost–benefit ratio of vigilance (Kavaliers and Choleris 2001). 'Giving-up-densities of food', i.e. the density of food at which an animal stops feeding or searching for food, has been used as an index of perceived risk of predation. If there is nutritious food around, it may be worth taking more of a risk than if the environment is barren (Miller 2002).

In severe PTSD it may seem that the cost–benefit analysis has broken down. The price that sufferers of PTSD pay for their hypervigilance is often tragic. Some turn their homes into fortresses, some seek geographical isolation, others seek both. Family life may be ruined, with resentment from partners and adolescent offspring at their seemingly ridiculously constricted lifestyles. Does this mean the theory breaks down? No. Remember a small dose of hypervigilance may be more obviously adaptive and that the genetic elements of the responses have largely been formed in ancestral times in environments bearing little resemblance to those of the developed nations in the twenty-first century.

Let us consider cost–benefit analyses in contemporary adolescents. Parents often wish that their adolescents would adjust their safety thresholds and become more alert to dangers – 'Please drive carefully', parents request. Youngsters prefer to have fun. Their priorities are social status and attraction; their parents' is their survival. Adolescents are in the mate-attracting stage of the life cycle. (In former times if they did not shortly secure a mate their personal survival would have been irrelevant from a gene's perspective.) Adolescents fear that if they routinely tell their friends to 'slow down', they will diminish their attractiveness. Valour, especially in males, has played an important role in demonstrating one's sexual worth in most mammalian species. What happens in adolescents who have accidents causing PTSD? They become more safety orientated and their social attractiveness to their peers may diminish, although I am not aware of any research that has examined this. This reasoning suggests that cost–benefit analyses may well be involved. A seriously threatening experience might force an adjustment of vigilance and defensive orientation despite the costs involved.

Let us turn to predation more specifically, remembering that according to the evolutionary theory, predation risk may have been the greatest selection pressure giving rise to defensive behaviours. The selection of anti-predator defence strategies requires vigilance in proportion to the risk, as determined by contextual analysis. Beyond vigilance, Vermeij's (1982) four-stage model of anti-predator strategies suggests that the first level defence is avoidance, which carries the cost of decreased access to resources such as food and mates. The second phase is recognition, or detection. Vermeij suggests that the third phase involves escape. This needs amending, as there should be provision for attentive immobility to assess the cost–benefit equations before expending energy on escape. Most of the cost–benefit research postdated Vermeij's work. Often prey can afford to defer flight or fight pending further risk assessment, so long as the predator is not within striking range. The fourth phase is subjugation or resistance, which I will cover in Chapters 8 and 9, as there is more to it than might be expected.

Predator avoidance involves outside or beyond visual field (or other sense) scenarios. The three remaining anti-predator responses are within visual field responses. I re-emphasize that predator avoidance and the remaining anti-predator mechanisms are under different selection regimes. The evolution of one regime reduces pressure on the other (Brodie et al. 1991). The evolution of a tortoise's shell eased the selection pressure on swift flight and aggression. PTSD cannot be a single genetic entity according to this reasoning. This suggestion is consistent with psychopharmacological research, which suggests a more heterogeneous PTSD symptom response profile to different antidepressants than is found in most other conditions for which these agents may be used (Davidson and van der Kolk 1996). Hence, predation studies suggest that safety and defence can be seen as two fundamental and separate information-organizing systems (Gray 1982, 1987; Gilbert 1993).

Detection of and response to threats rely more on fast control systems rather than slower cognitive systems. Detection of threats increases arousal and inhibits behaviour through what has been called the behavioural inhibition system. Its function is to stop behaviour that would lead to punishment or non-reward. The cue detection part of the system is located in a frontal-septal-hippocampal control system whereas the response output (flight/fight) is located in other limbic structures including the amygdala, ventromedial hypothalamus and central grey (Gray 1982, 1987).

Although not anatomically demonstrated, a behaviour safety system has also been proposed which is associated with rewarding emotions and the facilitation of behavioural exploration (Gray 1987; Gilbert 1993). The behavioural safety system involves slower reflective (cognitive) activity and the integration of information, in contrast to the affect-driven behavioural inhibition system.

Vigilance followed by safety signals deactivates defences. This is consistent with exposure therapies, which involve the sufferer confronting irrationally avoided behaviours for a sufficient period so that overarousal subsides. Someone with PTSD who avoids supermarkets may benefit from a carefully planned programme that involves visiting supermarkets. The lack of experience of the expected threats on so doing is associated with a reduction in future anxiety and irrational avoidance behaviours. In practice this is much more difficult than it sounds because of the resistance of PTSD responses to extinction (Mineka and Cook 1993).

Following a period of heightened risk of predation, a decrease in activity is observed in prey of most species (Lima 1998). Reduced activity may range from a few seconds in hermit crabs to several days in small mammals and is longer in more dangerous situations. Similarly, decreased activity is observed following a period of increased food availability. Resumption of activity is sooner in energy-depleted animals. Hunger pains might simply account for the earlier emergence of energy-depleted animals. However, it is also possible that fear of predators may be diminished in such states. I can think of at least one twenty-first century hominid, who, following vigorous exercise, worries less about perishables in his refrigerator that are past their 'use by' dates. His cognitions are, 'Too bad, I'm going to eat it anyway.' Anxiety/fear thresholds reflect ancestral survival issues and may be reset accordingly. Nature can motivate by decreasing fear as well as by increasing it. The possibility that hunger in humans in such contexts may reduce anxiety is undemonstrated but of potentially great importance, as we will shortly see.

Decreasing fear or choosiness also arises in other survival contexts. Female fish become less choosy regarding male partners in higher predation risk situations (Lima 1998; Crowley et al. 1991). I recall as a youngster being impressed by an observation from my butterfly collecting days. Seconds after I had placed my hapless victim in the killing jar, I noticed that in its death throes it expelled a gush of eggs. Presumably nature was gambling on a last ditch, 'What have you got to lose?' strategy. In times of war, humans of both sexes are known to behave more promiscuously. 'To hell with caution; I may not even be around to regret it!' is a common sentiment. This seems to reflect the observation of decreased choosiness of female fish under heightened risk of predation. It is consistent with both human cognitions and evolutionary logic.

If in times of threat individuals are less choosy regarding sexual partners, might the chronic overarousal of sexually abused persons with PTSD contribute to their often promiscuous behaviours? Repetition-compulsion involves a tendency for an abused person to re-enter or recreate potentially abusive situations. It is a useful *pattern level* description, but it fails to explain motivations. Could the heightened activation of defence systems in those chronically traumatized activate mechanisms that approximate these observations of fish? This would seem a potentially useful line of inquiry.

Another research question is what is the effect of pregnancy on pre-existing PTSD? Contrary to intuitive concerns about vulnerable pregnant ladies, in the animal world pregnancy has been found to be associated with pregnant females taking more risks than their stronger males, because of their increased need for nutrients (Miller 2002). Might the greater need for energy acquisition during human pregnancy reduce PTSD symptoms? Hiding away with PTSD would not have promoted healthy babies in ancestral times. Of course this may be a blind alley – but one remarkably easy to explore.

Similarly, energy-depleted animals are known to take greater risks with predators because of their need for food (Lima 1998). Nature could in theory promote this by both hunger pangs and by decreasing anxiety. Might energy depletion cause those with PTSD to experience a transient decrease in their symptoms? It would be both easy and interesting to conduct an experiment using fasting in PTSD patients. If a transient reduction in symptoms was noted, this might be thought worthless because of its transience. However, if there was support for this suggestion, fasting could be a useful adjunct to exposure therapies (Rothbaum, et al 2000). Exposure relies heavily on the concept of mastery – 'controllability' to the behaviourists – regaining power over fear that compromises lifestyle and self-identity. If the exposure task was to visit a supermarket or other public venue, it would be helpful to have an aid that increased the likelihood of experiencing success. Might conducting the exposure exercise in a hungry state – having missed a meal or two – increase success? Again the prospect seems unlikely, but this novel idea is another that would be remarkably easy to study. If it happened to be correct it would become a readily applicable adjunct in the treatment of a notoriously difficult disorder.

Such ecological cost–benefit research is unfamiliar to those in mental health. These preliminary suggestions are largely illustrative. I would be pleasantly surprised if pregnancy or hunger were associated with a reduction in symptoms. Nevertheless, this perspective of vigilance may lead to other discoveries.

A zonal approach to PTSD

Before examining the relevance of each mammalian defence to PTSD I will suggest a structure for approaching them. The determination of PTSD symptom profiles in individuals has received relatively modest attention to date. Could it be that symptom profiles are predictable, albeit in a diffuse and generalized way? If so, understanding the functions of defences and the contexts in which they arise may be important. This appears most evident for the contribution of appeasement to complex PTSD, as we will see in Chapter 8. However, it must be understood that any specificity between symptom profile and defences employed will be diffuse, as often more than one defence is relevant to the trauma which may 'itself' involve more than one trauma and be further influenced by the aftermath.

The importance of vigilance and risk assessment operating in conjunction with all the defences cannot be overstated. Further, vigilance combined with risk assessment are themselves defences. Radar, espionage and other military observation and intelligence constitute defensive activities involving vigilance and risk assessment. However, vigilance and risk assessment often indicate the need for more active defensive behaviours. Defence selection will also be influenced by contextual cost–benefit analyses.

PTSD may be usefully approached from the perspective of a zonal hierarchy of defences based on the distance of the potential victim from the source of the threat (Figure 6.1). Distance constitutes only one important determinant of defence selection. The capacity of the individual to deal with the threat by particular defensive strategies and cost–benefit analyses are also fundamental. The first level of defence from the zonal perspective is avoidance. This has also been described from a time-phase perspective as a pre-encounter defence (Nijenhuis et al. 1998). All the other defences are anti-predator strategies dependent on being within the field of the predator and so are under different selection pressures from avoidance, which is dependent on being outside this field (Brodie et al. 1991). These have also been described as post-encounter, circa-strike defences, which may then be followed by post-strike behaviour – the experience of pain and a period of recuperation (Nijenhuis et al. 1998).

Withdrawal and flight constitute the second defence from the zonal perspective. They are the first of the energy-expensive defence strategies, therefore will be employed much less frequently than avoidance, which has a more routine application. Flight is often combined with other strategies and in humans refuging is a key adjunct.

Aggressive defence is the third defence in the zonal sequence. In the context of a severe threat, aggressive defence will be selected when flight is unlikely to suffice. Aggressive defence is not synonymous with attack. Anger is an emotion with an exceptionally strong and effective signalling function (McGuire and Triosi 1998). Signalling

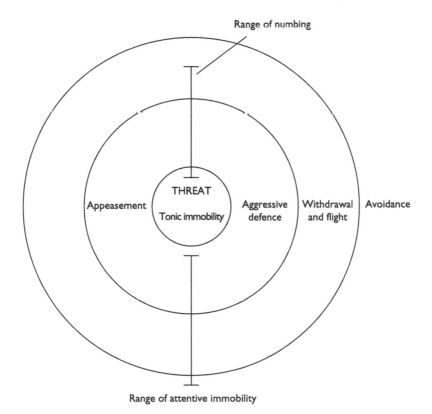

Figure 6.1 A zonal model of mammalian defences based on distance from the source of the threat

anger is associated with less risk of injury. In PTSD anger signalling is far more widespread and is employed earlier than actual attacking behaviour (see Chapter 7).

Attentive immobility crosses the boundaries of avoidance, withdrawal/flight, aggressive defence and appeasement. Two of its key functions are vigilance and risk assessment – but with a sense of urgency. An animal hears a noise and freezes. It may then return to feeding, reassured that its avoidance strategy is sufficient. Alternatively, it may freeze and then run, or realize it is trapped and will have to fight the predators. Freezing may also be a prelude to appeasement with conspecific aggressors if the power struggle is too one-sided and there is no opportunity for escape. Attentive immobility is transitional, serving often as a preliminary to other defences.

However, it also promotes inconspicuousness and signals threat or non-threat (preparedness to stand one's ground or disinclination to advance).

Immobility – attentive and tonic – cannot be seen as a single defensive entity. The two forms are controlled by different gene-neural processes and serve very different defensive functions.

The evolutionary chain of defences places numbing at the level of flight or beyond, as it is only relevant to engagement with the source of the threat. It has also been referred to as a circa-strike defence (Nijenhuis et al. 1998). Numbing is a state, not a behaviour, but clearly it is relevant to defence. Active flight and fight are both promoted if the prey is not distracted by pain. In contrast, following termination of an encounter the return of pain perception motivates recuperative behaviour, such as resting (Nijenhuis et al. 1998). Whether clinical numbing symptoms represent one broad category of defences is unclear, but opioid-mediated analgesia seems firmly established as one of its mechanisms (Miczec et al. 1982; Foa et al. 1992). Numbing symptoms may also be associated with appeasement and tonic immobility.

Appeasement lies beyond flight and aggressive defence in the zonal sequence. Appeasement implies the lack of opportunities for escape and entrapment by a dominant conspecific (Marks 1987).

Tonic immobility represents the last zonal defence, when all preferable alternatives have become irrelevant (Marks 1987; Ramos et al. 1999). It is activated by situations involving proximity to, or touch by the source of the threat, restraint and a sense of hopelessness. Rape and other civilian assaults involving these characteristics are contemporary acute contexts in which tonic immobility might be activated. Scenarios reflecting the original contexts may reactivate tonic immobility in chronic PTSD. For example, former rape victims may report freezing years later when their partners engage in unwelcomed rough sexual behaviour.

Avoidance

Avoidance combined with vigilance represents the first defence level against predators. Provided the costs are not excessive, staying away from predators is preferable to flight, which in turn is preferable to aggressive defence. Vigilance and risk assessment are inseparable from all of these strategies.

Vigilant avoidance was also the most widely utilized strategy early in our evolutionary history, because of reptilian energy limitations. Hence, it should have significant neurodevelopmental representation in the brainstem of our 'reptilian' brain. Sure enough the brainstem basal ganglia and extrapyramidal motor system control a number of automatic behaviours (MacLean 1949; Panksepp 1998, 2000). Paleomammalian and neomammalian elaborations have taken avoidance further as would be expected.

Avoidance behaviours might be expected to have a certain reptilian, automatic, unconscious quality. One early impression I had when I first started treating large numbers of people with PTSD was the 'mindless' quality of avoidance – much of it lying outside of awareness.

I recall a navy diver who as a result of war experiences had developed a phobia of the sea as one element of his broader PTSD. We agreed a homework task would be to walk towards, but not initially onto, a beach that he had not visited in years, despite it being nearby. When he had become confident with that, he would proceed with a series of stages approximating the end goal of paddling in the water. These plans were mutually agreed and it was clear that getting his feet wet was the final stage in the relatively distant future. He had no desire ever to swim again. For several months the results were the same. He would avoid commencing the exercises agreed to. He never was able to explain why, other than to say, 'I couldn't go in the water'. I would repeat the instructions, only to hear the same mystifying, 'I couldn't go in the water'.

This illustrates the *beneath awareness* reptilian quality at the heart of avoidance behaviours. The navy diver's avoidant behaviour appeared to come first, with words being subsequently found in attempts to rationalize the behaviour.

I will return later to vigilance and avoidance. First, let us consider the related defence – attentive immobility.

Attentive immobility

The consideration of immobility has been confused by the tendency to see immobility as a single entity with two faces – attentive and tonic. Immobility is not a single entity; it only masquerades as such. Attentive immobility is a transient hypervigilant state that keeps the head still for careful assessment of threat and reduces detection by others (Greene 1994). It can be viewed as vigilance on very high alert. The essential questions are how dangerous is the situation? Do I need to act definitively? Is flight possible or do I have to fight? Tonic immobility operates at the far end of the defensive spectrum (Marks 1987). It is a last-ditch resort, employed when escape is impossible and fighting is futile. It involves prolonged stillness and less physiological arousal. For now we will focus on attentive immobility.

Attentive immobility involves a frozen state of high arousal and is a prelude to more definitive prey decision-making (Lima 1998). It is another of the key mammalian defences, yet is not listed in the DSM-IV criteria. Might it be irrelevant, beyond the repertoire of symptoms experienced in PTSD? Might it be relevant, but because of its transitory nature considered unworthy of listing as a criterion?

Attentive immobility is a common symptom of PTSD despite not being listed as a criterion. It is unlikely to be volunteered as a symptom without specific inquiry. While its importance as a clinical symptom may be limited, its relevance is interesting. Attentive immobility serves a number of very short-term functions across a number of defence strategies. The assessment of whether energy should be expended on immediate flight or fight as opposed to ongoing vigilance often involves the 'better-safe-than-sorry' principle, which may coexist alongside cost–benefit considerations. The genetic ramifications of getting this wrong include immediate death versus less immediate starvation and/or reduced reproduction. The genes of animals getting the balance right will have been selected over evolutionary time. Attentive immobility is a component of selecting the correct response. In addition, when considering flight or fight, a burst of adrenaline assists preparation for this.

Attentive immobility occurs as a product of detection of a potential immediate threat, the distance between the subject and the threat and the escapability of the situation (Blanchard et al. 1991). The immediacy of the threat is a key aspect of freezing, startle and flight responses. Attentive immobility occurs across a range of defensive distances – from the antelope sniffing the air for a lion in the distance, to the rat cornered by a domestic cat. Defensive threat behaviours and overt attack in wild rats rise abruptly when the predator approaches the prey to within 1.0 or 0.5 metres defensive distance respectively (Blanchard et al. 1993). Startle also increases as a predator approaches suggesting an increase in muscle tension and readiness to react associated with freezing (Blanchard et al. 1991). When the situation permits escape, flight speed also increases with proximity of the predator.

Attentive immobility appears to be mediated by the lateral projections of the central grey, which also mediates stress-induced analgesia (Davis and Whalen 2001). The connections of the basolateral amygdala to the central nucleus of the amygdala, along with outgoing projections of the central nucleus, appear to collectively represent a central fear system involved in both the expression and acquisition of conditioned fear. Davis and Whalen (2001) in a scholarly neuroscientific review of amygdala functions suggest:

> An emphasis on the role of the amygdala in modulating moment-to-moment levels of vigilance in response to uncertainty has important implications for the study of human psychopathology. Hypervigilance is a key symptom of the anxiety disorders. Pathological anxiety may not be a disorder of fear, but a disorder of vigilance.

Their emphasis on vigilance as opposed to anxiety/fear is well taken.

Neurophysiology, diagnostic research tests and beyond

Systematic analysis of behavioural responses to ambiguous or potential threats remains in its infancy. Potentially, modern technology might assess vigilance and arousal phenomena as a diagnostic aid. Patients or research subjects could view a series of threat scenarios via video presentation. They would view provocative scenes, register their perceptions of threat and suggest their instinctive defensive responses. For example, a rape victim suffering PTSD while viewing ambiguous street scenes might suggest flight in less threatening scenarios than non-traumatized individuals. Physiological indices such as pulse and galvanic skin conductance as used in anxiety research might complement this. One of the problems with diagnosing PTSD is the variance in interpretations of the criteria, which are far from unambiguous. Potentially, such standardized approaches might become both practical and objective qualitative and quantitative diagnostic aids.

Vigilance literally means watchfulness. Might individuals with PTSD scan their environments more than those unaffected? I have not observed PTSD patients scanning for dangers within the safety of my consulting room, but some assure me they do so in other environments. Their lack of scanning in consultations may relate to their interacting with individuals (therapists) who present the combination of validating the sufferer's sense of threat, while signalling no threat. If so, there is a clear message here for family support.

A low threshold for visual scanning associated with PTSD might conceivably be objectively investigated under the above provocative and standardized video testing conditions. Might there be not only increased eye movements in those with PTSD, but also perhaps a characteristic pattern of eye movements difficult to feign, but amenable to analysis? If such ideas were to turn out to be correct, videotaped assessment of eye movements as a measure of vigilance, supported by a suitable computerized analysis could be of great use in research, clinical and medico-legal investigations.

Video and computerized eye-scanning movement tests may or may not turn out to be useful. An extension of this speculation, again involving eye movements, is so intuitively appealing from the evolutionary perspective that I will mention it despite the dubious odds of it being correct. Some orientation first is needed. There is a recent, popular, bizarre and widely used treatment for PTSD, the efficacy of which awaits clarification. Research conclusions are less than totally convincing (Chemtob et al. 2000) but many clinicians, even respectable ones, have confidence in the treatment. However, placebo and non-specific treatment effects contribute to the success rates of all psychotherapies, so it is easy to draw false conclusions from clinical impressions. On the other hand, clinical impressions may sometimes outperform objective research, which may lack the statistical power to demonstrate the effectiveness of treatments with relatively low, but genuine efficacy.

The treatment I refer to is known as 'eye movement desensitization and reprocessing' (EMDR). The procedure involves instructing the patient with PTSD to imagine a disturbing image associated with a traumatic memory, while tracking the clinician's finger or other visual stimulus that is quickly moved back and forth across the patient's visual field (Chemtob et al. 2000). This is used with some variations, until the patient's distressing cognitions have been replaced by more relaxed and adaptive ones. The consensus is that the procedure works, but that it may be essentially an exposure therapy in imagination, with the eye movements contributing little or no benefit.

Francine Shapiro, the pioneer of EMDR, has attempted to set the record straight about what were the components of EMDR. Shapiro (1999) described eight phases of treatment, which I will not reiterate as they are not particularly revealing. However, she clearly described various non-specific components common to all well-practised therapies, for example, careful assessment and rapport building. Exposure also is an important element, being administered gradually by way of desensitization combined with 'installation' of positive cognitions. Pathological sensations are targeted and mastery is promoted. All this is the stuff of everyday PTSD therapy, quite apart from anything to do with eye movements.

Shapiro's coverage of actual eye movements is less than revealing about the source of their beneficial effects. She volunteers: 'the use of eye movements in EMDR was based upon an accidental discovery of their apparent ability to defuse negative emotions and cognitions, rather than the logical outcome of a theoretical position.' She also notes that others have found 'that spontaneous eye movements are associated with unpleasant emotions and cognitive changes.' She does not clarify the direction of this association – i.e. whether eye movements cause or reflect unpleasant feelings.

If eye movements are an important and effective component of the EMDR result, might vigilance have something to do with it? Highly vigilant animals as I have suggested may scan their environment repeatedly while in a state of high arousal. Classical conditioning effects might result in a learnt association of eye-scanning movements and defensive tension. Perhaps massed practice of extreme scanning movements while visualizing the trauma in a reassuring atmosphere devoid of anxiety-provoking stimuli might be the therapeutic mechanism? Might it be that EMDR represents an exposure therapy akin to repeatedly and exhaustively scanning the environment for predators or hostile conspecifics and finding no threat there? This would seem an unusually plausible explanation for a seemingly highly improbable therapy.

Conclusions

The ethological concept of vigilance has much to offer to the study of PTSD. Vigilance is involved in all behavioural defences. Defences will be selected according to risk assessments and contextual analysis on the basis of cost–benefit ratios. A chain or sequence of defences can be useful for considering these issues. Generally avoidance will be the first line defence and potentially less costly than more active defences. The avoidance criteria of DSM-IV confuse true avoidance, flight and numbness, which are separate entities.

Defensive immobility has two components, attentive and tonic, serving very different functions controlled by different gene-neural processes. Attentive immobility may be viewed as a very transient but extreme state of vigilance promoting rapid and definitive defensive action.

The pressures of energy depletion and pregnancy may influence risk-taking. The possibility needs to be explored that such states might be associated with a reduction in fear facilitating the required risk-taking. If this were so, fasting might be a useful adjunct to exposure therapies. Although speculative, vigilance phenomena may present new avenues for investigating, diagnosing and treating PTSD sufferers.

Chapter 7

He who fights and runs away . . .

Withdrawal, aggressive defence and numbing

> He that is soon angry dealeth foolishly . . .
>
> Proverbs, The Bible

Withdrawal

We have seen that even unicellular organisms may learn withdrawal or flight responses and that predation pressure may have driven the early development of multicellularity, a process taking over 1000 million years – more than half the duration of life on earth (Stearns and Hoekstra 2000). Withdrawal had evolved further by the reptilian era, albeit reptiles did not have the flight capacity of mammals. We have established that withdrawal is under a different selection regime from avoidance (Brodie et al. 1991). A PTSD sufferer may avoid supermarkets. If pressured to override such avoidance, approach is often followed by flight. Hence, in clinical practice avoidance is the more common complaint. This mirrors the cost–benefit analyses discussed earlier (Vermeij 1982; Lima and Dill 1990; Lima 1998), whereby avoidance is usually less costly in terms of energy expenditure (and embarrassment) than flight. PTSD sufferers invited to confront certain of their avoidance behaviours often respond, 'It's not worth the hassle', a cost–benefit statement.

I have discussed the humble supermarket with Vietnam veterans who previously coped better with jungle warfare than they do now with the shopping trolley. Many simply will not enter supermarkets. I have asked what do supermarket aisles in particular suggest to these veterans? They often associate them with a specific sense of threat. Their *feelings* are that to enter an aisle involves trapping themselves in a tunnel of conspicuousness with no cover. Advancing or retreating would be associated with obvious vulnerability, should a threat appear at the far end. Of course cognitively they know the probability of such an attack is virtually zero, but their feelings tell them otherwise. As is often the case in PTSD, when there is a contest between feelings and logic, feelings tend to win. Perhaps this is because paleomammalian feelings are usually supported by reptilian behaviours.

Flight involves predator or other threat detection before it can be activated. Ambiguous threats that evoke flight without specific sensory identification of the threat are associated with contextual cues. Youngsters messing about in a graveyard after dark may become spooked – 'I'm out of here!' may be their verbal response, with a feeling as if a predator is on their heels. Their unease is more complex than fearing a mere telling off by the caretaker. In PTSD a person fleeing a shopping centre has detected some sense of threat, even though it may be based on an association of shopping centre cues with those of the original traumatic environment. Unconscious cues may have been established through classical conditioning, often with the help of preparedness. PTSD sufferers following humiliating flight experiences often report, 'I don't know why – I just couldn't.'

Refuging

While flight is often conceived of as 'running away', there is much more to it than this. Evolutionary theory suggests that slow-moving hominids will be inclined to flee to nearby refuges. They may also use those refuges for avoidance. Up to the time of australopithecines with their lack of weapons, aggressive defence against large predators would have been almost futile. Avoidance and early flight to a refuge would have promoted survival better. Further, the selection of refuging as a defence would often have been combined with the need to appear inconspicuous, e.g. utilizing attentive immobility in order to blend in with the foliage. Often the predator triggering flight might not yet have located the potential hominid prey. A medically retired policeman with PTSD described to me that when in pub gardens he prefers to be seated so that he blends in with the foliage. The children's game of 'hide and seek' is an archetypal representation of the combination of refuging and inconspicuousness.

Staying put in refuges often follows a period of heightened predation threat (Lima 1998). Sure enough, in PTSD we see the same thing. Following feeling socially threatened PTSD sufferers shut themselves away not just till the 'threat' has gone, but for a longer period. Animals feeding under time-related variation in predation risk strive for optimal anti-predator behaviour across states of risk (Lima and Bednekoff 1999b). Similarly, PTSD sufferers often prefer to visit supermarkets (if at all) at off-peak times – consistent with the risk-allocation hypothesis.

Fish, aquatic insects, gastropods, crustaceans, rodents and ungulates have all been observed to use refuging (Miller 2002). This suggests that refuging is partly subcortically based (unconscious), again supporting the observation that PTSD sufferers often cannot understand their reasons for flight. However, as the immediate predecessors of primates did not rely as much on refuging, convergence seems also involved, whether at cortical or subcortical levels.

While in earlier times refuges may have been up a tree, nowadays they are the home. Almost invariably where it is physically possible, PTSD sufferers, when fleeing, prefer to flee to their homes. The only exception is where the home has been the source of the trauma. It might be thought that in modern life it could hardly be otherwise. This is not so. If someone suffers PTSD as a result of rape or other assault in public, and later sees someone in public who resembles their attacker, she/he might be safer fleeing to a busy public location than to their home. Their potential attacker might prefer to follow his victim to a more private place than risk an attack in public. However, flight to refuges has been strongly programmed over evolutionary time and generally flight home will be selected as the preferred flight response.

The fourth DSM-IV avoidance criterion (C4), 'markedly diminished interest or *participation* in significant activities', and the fifth (C5), 'feeling of detachment and estrangement from others', may at times reflect refuging more than those issues, including even numbing, that they appear to represent. Consider the following case:

A patient reports that since the onset of PTSD she hardly ever sees her former friends; she does not go to the gym (having been a regular) and she no longer meets friends for coffee. However, when a friend calls round to her home, she enjoys the interaction. Her participation in usual activities (e.g. gym) is reduced and she is socially estranged from most friends due to her need to feel safe by remaining at home – refuging – but her preference for avoiding friends is context dependent.

Nevertheless, it is common for refuging to coexist with genuine social avoidance (not wanting friends). Refuging represents both avoidance and withdrawal strategies. Not only may animals retreat to their burrows, but also they may be reluctant to emerge from them.

Some persons hiding away at home will also report a need to lock their windows and doors. This clinically might be considered as the 'hypervigilance' overarousal (D4) criterion of DSM-IV. Yet it may be another component of refuging. There is no point in a reptile sheltering in a crevice if the predator can reach it inside.

A further component of refuging is the preference of great apes to rely on group defence with trusted members, preferably kin (Wrangham and Peterson 1996). This appears to have been neglected in the PTSD literature. The following case illustrates this well.

> A male machine operator aged in his early thirties was investigating a suspicious smell at work when an explosion occurred, with his bearing the brunt of a steam and chemical blast. He feared that a much more serious explosion would follow and despite his substantial burns took the necessary action to secure the situation. Having done so, his workmates hosed him down in what he found to be a highly traumatic experience in which he feared he would die. Reluctance to leave his home was a marked component of his subsequent PTSD. However, this was combined with a profound need for family proximity. Despite having previously confidently worked for several years in the fishing industry, which involved long periods away from his family and very tough workmates, he now found himself crying if his wife left him at home alone. He remarked, 'I don't seem to trust anyone except my wife and children. . . . I don't feel comfortable around people I don't know. . . . My biggest fear is losing my kids.'

In times of threat the best chances of loyal support lie with kin. In addition, offspring also carry one's genes, which must be protected.

The concept of refuging provides a deeper understanding of avoidance/flight behaviours. In my experience patients readily relate to the concept and benefit from so doing. Some have responded, 'So I'm not going mad after all!'

Group size and individual defence

A phenomenon well studied by ethologists is group size effects on defence strategies. Australopithecines were vulnerable to predators including false sabre tooth cats, scimitar toothed cats, bear-like animals and the older versions of contemporary predators including lions, leopards, cheetahs and hyenas (Treves, in preparation). Early hominids lived in small groups of probably twenty to thirty mostly related individuals and only rarely encountered other conspecifics, due to low population densities and territoriality (Treves and Pizzagalli 2002). Diet also limited group size in our great ape ancestry. Early hominids' discovery of the value of tubers and how to dig for them may have enlarged their natural group size compared with their mainly fruit-eating chimpanzee relatives.

However, much vigilance in non-human primates is directed not outwards to the outsider or predator, but inwards to in-group conspecifics. This reflects competition over resources and mates, with the associated dominance struggles that may sometimes result in death. Females from the same primate group direct more visual attention towards their in-group enemies than their allies (Watts 1998). Subordinates direct more glances to associates than do dominants (Alberts 1994). In great apes, baboons and geladas, social standing and social skills are important for both mate attraction and resource acquisition (Strum and Mitchell 1987; Wrangham and Peterson 1996). The higher frequency of in-group conflict offsets the less dangerous individual exchanges. Nevertheless, conspecifics from outside the group are more likely to inflict harm (Treves and Pizzagalli 2002).

Humans like other social species are orientated to group living, gaining many advantages from mutual coexistence, including safety and more time for foraging, though at the cost of competition for local resources. If humans choose to opt out of group life, with few exceptions our genetic heritage will under the direction of 'response rules' activate psychobiological response patterns promoting return to the group (Wenegrat 1984; Gilbert 1992). Loneliness sets in. Similarly, most of us can probably recall at times being fed up with family members, wishing they would go away for a while. No sooner do they do so, than we miss them.

An important aspect of group living is the composition of the group. In particular how many and who? We have seen that the great apes favour small groups for inconspicuousness. Because villages may have thousands of individuals and cities may have millions, an illusion has been created suggesting that the natural group size of *Homo* is large. It is true that the September 11 2001 New York tragedy activated a cohesive city response. But sympathy was also activated globally and largely as a result of technology. These sympathies are associated with the 'idea' of the group, which has a story-using function. The more one identifies with it, the stronger the sympathy. The less we identify with those affected by tragedies, the less instinctive concern we feel. The western world's neglect of African health and economic problems is a product of indifference based on lack of identification. Concern for the well-being of those who are of no direct benefit to us is largely intellectually based. Our instincts are more orientated to resources and in-group out-group notions.

Early storytelling was dependent on word of mouth transmission. Writing and recent technology have permitted identification with very large groups. However, the true pre-civilization group size for humans was much smaller and associated with much stronger bonds. Great apes evolved with inconspicuousness and trust being high on their list of defensive strategies. Ancestrally, relatedness has been the best measure of trustworthiness. Police attending domestic disputes know to exercise caution rescuing the 'battered wife', for she may suddenly side with her brutal husband to attack the well-intentioned rescuer.

We have seen that widespread conspecific killing not only occurs in our chimpanzee relations, but also is much more common in contemporary hunter-gatherers than romantic notions have suggested (Wrangham and Peterson 1996). Conspecific killing is likely to have exerted substantial selection pressures, albeit probably only over a few to several million years. How might the hominid group size have been influenced by serious threats from within? Clues may be provided from the bonobo, the most peaceful of the non-human great apes, which has the largest group size and the almost solitary orangutan, which is the most violent. Serious in-group threats in hominids might have activated a tendency to retreat from a larger to a more closely related and therefore smaller group size. A strong leader would also help and might have partially offset this influence.

In modern PTSD reduced capacity to trust others is well recognized (van der Kolk 1996a) though not listed in the DSM-IV. It is associated with and promotes retreat to the nuclear family. Refuging would further drive this psychobiological response. This would be accompanied by signals to others to keep their distance. This strategy might be self-reinforcing as rapists and armed robbers invade one's home infrequently – creating an illusion that a relatively solitary existence is meeting the needs of defence.

Finally in relation to group size, it is intriguing that modern-day warfare has developed basic fighting units of ten men constituting sections, with three sections or thirty men forming a platoon. These group sizes are what have been suggested for early hominids. Might these defensive/offensive units have 'evolved' through military trial and error, settling on unit sizes for which we are genetically programmed? Raiding and very recent war-induced selection pressures would have been great. Of course there are other military unit sizes of much greater magnitude. However, the importance of group loyalty in great apes (except the orangutan) including contemporary humans is reflected in the training employed in these basic military units. It may go even deeper. In the Second World War the US military introduced a rapid replacement system whereby when a soldier from a section was killed or injured, he would be quickly replaced. The replacement would be an outsider who might even go into combat that day without recalling the names of his new 'brothers'. The psychiatric casualty rate in such replacements became so high that this otherwise highly efficient policy had to be abandoned (Shephard 2002). Furthermore, when section commanders were killed or wounded, the psychiatric casualty rate of survivors would suddenly rise. These military observations are consistent with what would be predicted from observations of non-human great ape group defences.

Aggressive defence

In contrast to avoidance and flight, aggressive defence is exclusively catered for in the DSM-IV by only one criterion, the second of the overarousal criteria (D2) – irritability or outbursts of anger. Irritability/anger is one of the most useful symptoms for discriminating PTSD from simple phobias and the other anxiety disorders, as none of these include anger as a feature. Abram Kardiner (1941) noted that in his opinion every traumatic neurosis involved aggressiveness.

However, how do we reconcile PTSD producing a retreat to the nuclear family and the high levels of aggression directed to family members? Is it just a generalization from hostility directed outside the family? I believe there is more to it.

Our understanding of aggression has been influenced by morality. Aggression is generally perceived as an unpleasant and undesirable phenomenon in our day-to-day existence. I have considerable sympathy for this perspective, but it neglects a vital function of aggression. Michael McGuire and Antonio Troisi (1998) in their text *Darwinian Psychiatry* review the key emotions, making an observation that I believe is so important and clearly expressed that I will quote it in full:

> Most important, the influence of anger on the behaviour of others cannot be too strongly underscored: Whatever else anger may be, it is one of the most effective ways of rapidly altering others' behaviour. Indeed, with the possible exception of intense pain, no other affect has such a predictable impact.

In other words, much of the function of anger is less about doing harm to others and more about influencing their behaviour to accord with one's own needs, or the needs of the other.

In PTSD much anger towards family members may be, from a modern perspective, a misguided attempt to protect family members. Turning one's home into Fort Knox and berating any lapses in high-security routines by family members is common in PTSD. Anger serves a signalling function and does so very effectively. Furthermore, the human brain is very highly developed with respect to the recognition of conspecific anger facial signals (Panksepp 1998).

Earlier I observed that it is curious that the word anger is routinely used to characterize human aggression, but not that of predators. Let us examine this more closely with respect to signalling. If a predator is stalking prey, what might it want to signal to its prey? Nothing at all. If it is detected the hunt may already be lost. The only signal that could conceivably be of use would be a deception signalling no threat. This does not preclude the possibility that anger signals at the very moment of striking might then reduce resistance. However, for most of the predation sequence anger would be a liability.

Might anger be mostly a human emotion? How might a prey animal respond to a predator at close quarters? When a dog corners a cat in an archetypal predator–prey scenario, the cat will make its fur stand on end and arch its back to increase its apparent size and hiss alarmingly. If it could talk, surely it would utter something angry and rude. Its behaviour serves exactly the signalling function to which we have just alluded. The dog may also be snarling but only as it is beyond the approach phase of the predation sequence and into the subjugation phase (Endler 1986).

PTSD may be induced by natural disasters. Anger signals and violent behaviour are of no use against a tornado. Might levels of anger in environmentally induced PTSD be less? Might this be a way of testing the theory that PTSD is based on an adaptive mechanism? Possibly, but the situation is complicated by secondary issues. The tornado may not respond to anger but family members do: 'For goodness sake get in that shelter quickly!' Nevertheless, broadly the evolutionary theory suggests that anger may be generally less in environmentally induced PTSD.

The mammalian defence model predicts that aggression will be mostly about signalling as opposed to violence, which even for fitter individuals carries unacceptably high risks for routine use. The greater use of aggression for signalling is reflected in PTSD. This does not mean violence does not occur in PTSD, as I was recently reminded.

I performed a medico-legal examination on a young man who had escaped virtually physically unscathed from a car accident in which the driver and another passenger were not so fortunate. His experience of the accident and its aftermath was about as bad as it can get. I will spare you the details. Since his trauma he had lost count of the number of people he had uncharacteristically assaulted – mostly strangers who looked at him the wrong way. Despite my seeing him at the request of his solicitor, from the outset of the interview I was highly aware of signals indicating that I might be attacked. It was an unfortunate reality that the interview could not avoid touching exquisitely sensitive issues. With my blessings he left the consulting room on two occasions to settle himself down, no doubt with his generous consideration of my welfare. On his second return I offered him the option of adjourning the interview until another time. He indicated he wished to get it over with, but requested that we continue it in the car park where he could smoke and be unconfined. For the first time in my career I performed the remainder of a now slightly more relaxed but formal interview sitting on a low wall carefully out

of arm's reach. At the end of this traumatic experience, as he
was about to leave, the young man extended his hand. We
shook hands with a mutual signalling of gratitude, too complex
for words to describe.

Such experiences remind me that my paleomammalian brain is alive
and well, and why I chose psychiatry as a career. Nevertheless, I am
glad that my office usually suffices.

Numbing

Unlike the mammalian defensive behaviours I have discussed, numbing is not a behaviour, it is a physiological process or state. There are
other physiological states involved in defence and PTSD, such as a
quickening of the heart rate, increased muscle tension and so on. I
will address numbing only, as numbing symptoms are found and
confused in the DSM-IV's 'avoidance' criteria (C4, C5 and C6) (Foa
et al. 1992) and much might be learnt by clarification and further
study of numbing phenomena.

The definition and range of numbing symptoms in PTSD remain
unclear. Words can mislead, and the main reasons I use the term
numbing is that everybody else does and alternatives have not been
introduced. From an evolutionary perspective, numbing probably
represents defences further on from avoidance. It would be unnecessary to experience opioid-mediated analgesia unless engagement with
a threat has occurred. It is much more relevant to flight, aggressive
defence and beyond, whereby distraction by pain might prove fatal.

In acutely hazardous situations such as combat, becoming emotional over the loss of comrades may increase the risk to oneself.
Detachment may promote survival. Most would agree that ongoing
loss of capacity for loving feelings would constitute emotional numbing. The opioid-mediated analgesia associated with defeat is another
example of numbing. Whether these types of numbing arise from a
single entity, or whether they arise from different gene-neural processes is unclear. Opioid activity facilitates defence under attack, by
way of pain suppression (van der Kolk 1996c). However, the person
in the midst of attack who does not feel his wounds may be far from
emotionally numb, although I concede that warm feelings for others
would not be his preoccupation.

It is common for clinicians to hear of seriously injured people who when attacked had fought back or run away, only to collapse with the onset of severe pain, on reaching safety.

I recall a man who illustrates this well. He was a victim of two assaults in quick succession in public and by the same unknown assailant. Having floored his assailant for the second time in an hour, he wondered why someone with such inferior fighting skills would return a second time for more punishment. As he left the scene he noted a sticky sensation under his shirt. The multiple puny 'punches' to his trunk he had felt prior to flooring his attacker the second time had in reality been multiple life-threatening stab wounds. Shortly after, he endeavoured to calm the nearby police, who were horrified by his blood loss. He described fearing his own demise while struggling to stay conscious long enough to receive appropriate assistance. Although he recovered from his physical wounds, he developed PTSD.

This example of course portrays a single and acute form of opiate-mediated numbing. Under extended combat conditions, protracted stress reactions may become so overwhelming that a soldier's judgement is affected and he may dissociate pain, horror and grief to such an extent that his behaviour is grossly impaired. This numbing may in part represent yielding behaviour or learned helplessness (Solomon et al. 1996; Shephard 2002).

Some data suggest that the best predictors of severity of later emotional numbing are problems with hyperarousal at the time of the acute event (Litz and Gray 2002). Paradoxically, this represents an acute excess of feelings leading to a chronic deficiency of them.

Repeatedly attacked mice have been found to show decreased pain perception to heat applied to their tails, suggesting endogenous opioid-mediated analgesia activated by stress such as defeat (Miczec et al. 1982). Rats subjected to territorial defeat may display reduced serum antibodies (Fleshner et al. 1989). In humans with PTSD, low levels of emotional expression have been found to lead to impairment of immune function and the development of illness. Human victims of repeated traumas display fewer numbing symptoms than those with single traumas (Foa et al. 1992). This parallels the analgesic experiences of repeatedly defeated rodents. Detachment, constricted affect and decreased interest in activities are highly prevalent in the repeatedly abused, who also experience more amnesia and dissociation.

Emotional numbing is considered one of the most intractable symptoms of PTSD. Furthermore, it is less intermittent than re-experiencing symptoms, anxiety and irritability. Fluoxetine has a particularly beneficial effect on the numbing of PTSD (Davidson and van der Kolk 1996). This is curious as while fluoxetine works primarily on serotonergic pathways, numbing primarily involves dopaminergic pathways (Bremner et al. 1999). However, if emotional (as opposed to opiate-mediated) numbing is really a form of yielding, fluoxetine would be expected to help reverse this more depressive response.

Borderline personality disorder, which is related to chronic PTSD, often results from repeated childhood sexual abuse and has a strong association with numbing. The disorder is characterized by chronic anger, sense of alienation and self-destructive behaviour, commonly by repeated self-cutting and self-inflicted cigarette burns. Self-mutilation is often associated with relief of emotional tension and dissociation is commonly involved. Again endogenous opioids are thought to mediate this analgesia (van der Kolk 1996a).

Hence, opiate-mediated analgesia seems clearly adaptive in the context of acute physical defence. It also is associated with chronic PTSD. However, the emotional constriction that is also found in PTSD may have more in common with chronic withdrawal (flight) and yielding phenomena than with aggressive defence. Research on lack of controllability and predictability and learned helplessness suggests these experimental paradigms are effective inducers of numbing symptoms, although it is less certain as to whether the different symptoms are part of a single phenomenon (Mineka and Hendersen 1985). If numbing does represent a range of phenomena we may need to use terms that reflect this.

Conclusions

Flight is a defence observed from unicellular organisms through to the most complex animals. Flight is an energy-expensive defence strategy; therefore it is employed less frequently than avoidance, which has a more routine application. Flight is often combined with other strategies and in humans and other great apes refuging and group defence relying on close relationships are the key adjuncts. This goes some way to explaining why sufferers of PTSD retreat to their homes, are reluctant to come out and may rely excessively on their families.

Aggressive defence involves at least two strategies – violence and much more commonly, signalling. Anger is an emotion with an exceptionally strong and effective signalling function. Anger is not the same as aggression. Aggressive predators stalking prey do not benefit by advertising their approach. Anger is more commonly of use to potential prey and conspecifics. The evolutionary theory of adaptiveness suggests that context would be important for symptom development. A trauma evoked in a context appropriate to the expression of anger, for example a personal assault, might be expected to generate more problems with excessive anger than one in which anger signalling would be futile, such as many natural disasters. The term 'aggressive defence' accommodates both the widely used angry signalling and the much more costly fight responses. However, the signalling aspect lies earlier in the defensive sequence. There are important contextual differences relevant to the activation of these two aggressive defence components and there may be important differences in terms of neurophysiology.

Numbing symptoms are located in the 'avoidance behaviours' of DSM-IV. The evolutionary chain of defences suggests that opiate-mediated numbing would belong substantially later than true avoidance, with it being more relevant to engagement with the source of the threat, activating effective flight or fight. Acute versus chronic perspectives and deficient terminology confound the concept of numbing. Whether numbing symptoms represent one broad category of defences remains unclear, but opioid-mediated analgesia seems firmly established as one of its mechanisms.

Chapter 8

The paradox
of appeasement

> The most disadvantaged peace is better than the most just war.
> Deciderius Erasmus, *c.* 1466–1566

A hidden problem

Appeasement is comprised of elements of pacification, conciliation and submission. It is one of the key mammalian defences, and one about which I have said little so far. If PTSD is an overactivation state of human and other animals' defensive strategies, there is no reason why a major strategy should be omitted. An evolutionary theory that does not include all the key defences is highly suspect, in my opinion, or is at least missing something.

The apparent lack of coverage of this phenomenon reflects the traditional conceptualization of PTSD. It is not just the DSM-IV that has slept on appeasement; psychiatry in general has failed to adequately recognize it. In a recent, leading and very comprehensive textbook of psychiatry (Sadock and Sadock 2000), with an index a staggering 21,560 column centimetres long, the word 'appeasement' is not listed. Far from being rare in traumatized individuals, I suggest that appeasement is widespread in clinical practice, is most definitely part of the evolutionary theory and is fundamental to some types of PTSD.

Appeasement functions

Appeasement is primarily a defence strategy relevant only to conspecifics and mostly confined to social species including our own. It is an almost totally irrelevant defensive response to predators.

Accordingly, it stands in contrast to all the other mammalian defences in which predation threat figures prominently. The association of appeasement with socialization suggests that it is likely to involve greater components of neomammalian selection pressures, than the other defences.

When withdrawal (flight) and aggressive defence are not viable defensive responses to conspecifics at close range, appeasement may be the preferred option. Appeasement involves a subordinate interacting with a dominant individual. If leaving the group is a legitimate option, appeasement may be unnecessary. Withdrawal may be sufficient. Appeasement is a defensive strategy utilized when the subordinate or potential victim has to remain in proximity to the threatening dominant individual(s). The complex group social structures of most primate species often require defeated and/or subordinate members to remain within the group, to avoid isolation and the associated predation risk (Wrangham and Peterson 1996). This effectively precludes flight other than to the periphery of the group (Gilbert 1992).

John Price and colleagues (2004) have described the evolutionary relevance of appeasement to depressive, anxiety and somatization disorders. In a close encounter with a conspecific group member, where flight is not an option, the choices may be viewed as escalation or de-escalation. The former involves fighting and the possibility of winning, but involves an escalation of costs associated with losing. De-escalation involves appeasement behaviours signalling, 'I am no threat.' While appeasement may be a social defence with considerable neomammalian contributions, it is still represented in the three triune brain levels. With depression the reptilian component of appeasement is associated with signalling to no one in particular a state of general debility. This will be accompanied by paleomammalian feelings and neomammalian cognitions, with associated signals directed at the dominant individual(s) (Price et al. 2004).

Conspecific confrontations may activate feelings of shame in the subordinate. However, if the confrontation involves greater inequality and threat, fear may dominate. Curiously, shame has been relatively neglected by researchers and clinicians, in part because of patients' reluctance to divulge it (Gilbert 1992). Shame is an emotion that is so uncomfortable to the self that dissociation is often involved when it emerges in the context of PTSD (van der Kolk and McFarlane 1996). Shame is common in rape victims who not only experience horror, but also may blame themselves for their humiliation. It also arises in the context of survivor guilt, in which individuals feel guilty for surviving traumas when others did not (Aarts and Op den Veld 1996).

A context for fear-based appeasement

Most of us have childhood memories of being caught out by a superior figure, having committed some wrong-doing. The challenge was to figure out the best appeasement strategy. Escalating the confrontation with the dominant school principal was not an option. Note that in this scenario we would have felt both fear and shame.

Primates, including baboons and macaques, have been observed to be defeated and retreat, only to then return to their dominant and protest until some sign of acceptance is received (Chance 1988). This phenomenon is referred to as 'reverted escape'. It is a paradoxical defence as it involves escaping *to* not *from* the aggressor. The dominant, having accepted the subordinate back, may later repeat threatening behaviour causing further arousal and reverted escape, which consolidates the dominant/subordinate orientation and the associated bond. Thereby this paradoxical bond is maintained over long periods.

Primatologist Frans de Waal (1988) noted that male hamahydras baboons herd their females by neck bites, which results in reverted escape by the females. He notes that a number of researchers including the pioneer of ethology, Konrad Lorenz, have suggested that aggression might have a positive influence on bonding under some circumstances. Social structures are more stable if there is acceptance of the 'pecking order'. This raises the prospect that violence under some specific circumstances may strengthen group cohesion. Adolf Hitler was evil personified, but he successfully fostered national cohesion. Attempts at appeasement may have been the foundations of the Jewish response to his cruel authority, although many other factors, including the lack of feedback about the results of appeasement attempts by others, would have been involved. While it is possible that violent dominants may at times foster group cohesion, generally better-functioning affiliative social groups will interact by friendly gestures, cooperation and other non-violent peace-promoting behaviours.

The Stockholm syndrome

Let us briefly go back in time a few million years. Early hominids lived in groups of around twenty to thirty individuals. They rarely came in contact with other groups (with hostile interactions being the rule on so doing). A subordinate would rarely have had the luxury of defection. It is likely that on the odd occasion that a female moved to another group, this may have been involuntary and associated with ongoing subordination, including forced intercourse with males and violent resentment from other females. Subordinate exiled males may have fared even worse. Hence, to stay with its group a humiliated subordinate hominid had to make peace with the more dominant individuals. Signalling to the dominants how abhorrent their behaviours were would not have helped; signals of humility would.

Returning to more recent times, in 1973 a robbery in a bank in Stockholm resulted in four hostages being held captive for around six days (Strentz 1979). Interviews with the former hostages and observations of their behaviour following being freed revealed the paradoxical development of positive feelings in the hostages towards their captors, and to a lesser extent positive feelings in their captors towards their hostages. This phenomenon became known as the 'Stockholm syndrome'. The former hostages defended their captors and condemned the police who rescued them. One of the female captives became intimately involved with her captor and later became engaged to him.

In another incident, criminals discovered an undercover police agent in their midst. The leader set about escaping, leaving instructions that the agent be killed, if he (the leader) did not phone in to confirm his successful escape. The phone call followed and the agent lived. Subsequently the agent hesitated to testify against the leader, even several years later, feeling that the leader had saved his life (Kuleshnyk 1984).

In hostage situations police authorities consider the development of the Stockholm syndrome to be desirable, as it serves a protective function. Its desirability is all the more surprising, as there are significant negatives associated with the syndrome. Police may no longer be able to trust hostages in prolonged sieges and former hostages may be unreliable witnesses (Turco, (1987). The development of the Stockholm syndrome requires a significant passage of time. There is disagreement among police over whether incidents should be deliberately prolonged to allow time for the syndrome to develop; however, it is accepted that the longer the siege, the more likely it is that the syndrome will develop (Kuleshnyk 1984). While prolonged sieges are dangerous and traumatic, the Stockholm syndrome increases the chances of the captives emerging alive.

Potential explanations proffered for the Stockholm syndrome have included the captors' meeting the hostages' needs for food, medicines and so forth, with the hostages identifying with their dominant captors as a child might identify with a parent – regression plus identification with the aggressor (Kuleshnyk 1984). Hostages may subconsciously and consciously recognize that behaving cooperatively and pleasantly with their captors may be advantageous. In some circumstances the captives may come to believe in their captors' cause. However, symptomatically former hostages may develop startle reactions, phobias, night sweats and other symptoms of PTSD.

Auerbach et al. (1994) tested the Stockholm syndrome within the context of interpersonal theory. Interpersonal variables generally have a circular structure organized around two central dimensions of, first, control (dominance–submission), and second, affiliation (friendliness–hostility). This concept was upheld in an experiment using simulated captivity. The less the 'hostages' perceived the simulated terrorist as dominant and the more they perceived him as friendly, the better was the hostage adjustment. Also the more the terrorist perceived hostages as friendly, the more positive was the experience for hostages.

Favaro et al. (2000) conducted the first study of trauma in kidnap victims in Sardinia, Italy. Kidnapping in Sardinia is common, and was associated with a 21 per cent mortality rate for the period 1960–1980. Rates of PTSD and major depressive disorder were extremely high, 45.9 and 37.5 per cent respectively, and generally similar to those associated with concentration camps and torture. They also found that the number of humiliating and deprivation experiences predicted the development of the Stockholm syndrome, but not PTSD or major depressive disorder. Contrary to earlier suggestions, they found the use of violence did not prevent the reaction.

Perhaps the most famous kidnapping in this context was that of Patty Hearst in 1974 by the Symbionese Liberation Army (SLA). Following her kidnapping she was confined over many months, debased, raped, tortured and forced to participate in lawbreaking, including the infamous bank robbery for which she would later be convicted. She would publicly decry her family and fiancé, and praise the SLA (Weed 1976). Her first identity change was an enforced one, to *Tania*, but following additional trauma she developed a dissociative pseudo-identity, *Pearl*, along with other symptoms of PTSD (West and Martin 1994). The conventional psychiatric explanation for her apparent defection to the enemy is 'identification with the aggressor'. This explanation provides a *How?* answer, but not really a *Why?* Identification with the aggressor is an intrapsychic defence mechanism. All intrapsychic defences fulfil the functions of reducing distress, but as an answer to *why* she acted so out of character over long periods, this explanation seems lacking. Others have described her as having been 'brainwashed'. Brainwashing usually involves a captive being repeatedly forced under threat of death or other grave consequences, to confess their inferior and shameful status. The escape from this torture is to become compliant and to side with the captors. At a fundamental mammalian defence selection level, the appeasement survival instinct provides a greater understanding for Patty Hearst's 'bizarre' psychological and behavioural defection to her enemies.

Current knowledge of terrorism reactions can assist the understanding of some forms of child abuse reactions. The child, like the hostage, commonly turns to and accepts the explanations of the abuser. The child views herself as bad and deserving of punishment. In discussing these phenomena Goddard and Stanley (1994) noted that the child's protecting role towards the abusive adult has never been adequately explained. I suggest appeasement appears to meet this need.

Complex PTSD

Judith Herman (1992) touched on these issues from a traditional phenomenological perspective in a landmark paper. She noted that 'prolonged, repeated trauma can occur only where the victim is in a state of captivity, unable to flee, and under the control of the perpetrator.' She described the result as 'Complex PTSD', which I described in Chapter 2. She noted a number of major contributors to the field of PTSD have suggested the notion of a spectrum of PTSDs. Compared with ordinary PTSD, complex PTSD involves more complex, diffuse and tenacious symptoms, characteristic personality changes, and vulnerability to repeated harm, both self-inflicted and at the hands of others. Three commonly observed categories of symptoms not readily catered for by the DSM-IV, include somatization (the expression of distress through bodily symptoms), dissociation, and affective changes, particularly depression. Ethological ranking theory of anxiety and depression resulting from involuntary subordination (Gilbert 1992) concurs with this. Herman (1992) noted, 'To the chronically traumatized person, any independent action is insubordination, which carries the risk of dire punishment.'

Different mammalian orders manifest different submissive behaviours. Many reduce their apparent size. Even humans cower. Dogs may submit by way of infantile mimicry, rolling on their backs like puppies. Primates often use a sexual strategy. Not only females, but also submitting adult male primates may behave like females offering their genital regions to the dominant male, which might respond by emphasizing its status by token mounting actions (Kummer 1995; Price et al. 2004). In humans this expression of dominance is frequently encountered in particularly violent closed subcultures such as prisons and sometimes the armed forces. Newcomers may be sodomized as a means of promoting submission, acceptance of subordinate status and of the group's codes of conduct.

Sexual abuse of young children and of 'battered wives' may at times be associated with degrees of compliance that seem paradoxical to our civilized minds. The compliance is a form of reverted escape (Chance 1988) fulfilling the function of appeasement. As observed in primates, a sexual offering may appease the dominant individual. Even adult stalking victims may at times 'consent' to sexual intercourse with their stalkers in desperate attempts to pacify them. However, submitting humans may use diverse and flexible behavioural strategies including shrinkage in size, infantile and sexual behaviours as suits the situation. Culture may further ritualize such behaviours (Price et al. 2004).

In humans repetition-compulsion later in life may transform the original victim into the perpetrator of similar offences (van der Kolk 1989). The abusive behaviour by the abused is said to represent a defence against feelings of vulnerability, or identification with the aggressor. This psychoanalytic explanation is from an intrapsychic perspective. From behavioural, interpersonal and ecological perspectives, I suggest it also represents and signals an attempt to establish higher status, utilizing their familiarity with appeasement to demand submission from others. Similarly, familiarity with appeasement seems relevant to explaining why some abused women may move from one abusive relationship to the next.

Herman (1992) suggested that repetition-compulsion phenomena 'are not simple reenactment or reliving experiences. Rather, they take a disguised symptomatic or characterological form.' Such a description does not actually contribute much to understanding these phenomena. She is generous with phenomenological labels that do not contribute much to understanding. I quote Herman, 'Earlier concepts of masochism or repetition-compulsion might be more usefully supplanted by the concept of a complex traumatic syndrome.' At the time of writing this in 1992 her suggestion was useful. There were a number of contemporary overtly political, but largely justified sentiments in her paper, which amount to 'Stop blaming victims, understand their experiences instead' (my words). I fully support this, but suggest that understanding repetition-compulsion involves both recognizing the *pattern* of repetition-compulsion and its underlying social ranking function, that of upgrading an individual's subordinate status by activating appeasement behaviours in other subordinate individuals – often children for obvious reasons.

Conclusions

An evolutionary theory of fear-based traumatic psychological states should encompass all the fundamental mammalian defence strategies. If PTSD is accepted as a disorder of defensive functioning some provision for appeasement-related symptoms would seem necessary. Psychiatry has neglected appeasement as a phenomenon despite the growing recognition of the need to cater for complex PTSD, which I suggest might be conceptualized as a disorder of appeasement. Prisoners of war, hostages, kidnap victims, stalking victims, battered partners and sexually abused children commonly employ this defence. Appeasement offers an explanation for the mechanism underlying complex PTSD and supports it as an entity. At first glance appeasement might seem maladaptive, but in less civilized times would have been protective. Appeasement responses are highly context dependent, supporting the suggestion that PTSD generally may be adaptive *and* maladaptive, as opposed to purely pathological.

Chapter 9

A last resort
Tonic immobility

> the demeanor of the figure, rushing hurriedly through my brain, had paralyzed – had chilled me into stone. I stirred not – but gazed upon the apparition. There was a mad disorder in my thoughts – a tumult unappeasable.
>
> Edgar Allan Poe, 1809–1849

Desperate measures

Tonic immobility is the final defence in a chain of anti-predator responses involved in maintaining survival (Ramos et al. 1999). It involves a temporary profound state of motor inhibition. It may be activated by proximity to the threat, restraint or other physical contact between predator and prey, in situations appearing hopeless. In some species, such as sharks, turning the animal upside down may induce it. Turning these vertebrates upside down also results in their becoming long-sighted in trance-like states (Hueter et al. 2001). This is very different from attentive immobility associated with highly vigilant risk assessment, with options including flight and counterattack. These two forms of immobility are different evolutionary phenomena masquerading under an illusion of similarity.

Prey about to be consumed by a predator may have some last-ditch tricks in reserve. Ceasing struggling may confuse the predator, fail to activate the killing reflex and also involves pretending to be a noxious threat – involuntary defecation may assist this. Tonic immobility is a primitive mechanism that is predominantly reflexive, although it can be mimicked cognitively, as known to hikers when bears and human paths cross. The reflex nature of tonic immobility is illustrated by the fact that it may persist beyond the period of threat, as in humans who remain frozen with fear well after the threat has passed. The particularly strong Todesstellreflex in chickens in this state may even prove fatal (Dixon 1998).

Rape victims at times report having been paralysed with fear. The potential traumatic triggers of 'predator' proximity, physical contact with the 'predator' and restraint are all elements of the rape context. However, there can be alternative explanations for non-resistance in rape, including attentive immobility involving weighing up the risks of fighting back, looking for an opportunity to flee and even a conscious decision to accept the humiliation to promote survival (a form of appeasement). Prolonged immobility, extending beyond the duration of the assault, is more consistent with tonic immobility.

> A young woman with PTSD described to me having been alone attending a café early one morning when two male robbers sprung up in front of her behind the counter. One brandished a knife and the other struck her. She froze and remained in this immobile state for some minutes after their departure before she could call for help.

Tonic immobility is an objective behavioural description of experience. What might be the subjective perspective of the victim? The victim is paralysed with fear yet still fully 'conscious'. The mind is aware but overwhelmed, unable to initiate voluntary movements. Their inner selves would seem to be split – in some form of dissociation.

While acute traumatic experiences are most typical of tonic immobility, the following case illustrates how it can occur in PTSD.

> The young woman I described above, who developed PTSD following being held up at knifepoint in the café, had another later episode of tonic immobility. Approximately one year after the robbery she experienced problems with her partner's brother, who had previously made her feel intimidated. Recently, he and his partner angrily entered her home when she was alone, believing she had sold some of his possessions that he had lent her. He barged past her and opened a cupboard where his gear should have been, to find it was still there – as she had told him.

He then calmed down slightly, but continued to be critical. My patient recounted how during this incident she had frozen and found herself unable to speak for two minutes, most of which was after the cupboard had been opened. Subsequently, she was more reluctant than unable to speak for a further ten minutes. During the initial two-minute speechless state she felt overwhelmed by fear and flashbacks of her café knife-wielding assailants, barely attending to what was occurring in her home. She volunteered, 'It was like I was in two places at once.' She had wanted to speak up for herself in her home but words would not come. Other key aspects of the incident were feeling her sanctuary had been invaded and having nowhere to flee to (compare refuging). In addition the male had brushed against her aggressively and she was confined in a room close to the source of her threat.

Hysteria or PTSD?

Dramatic descriptions of traumatic immobility states are to be found in accounts of the two world wars (Shephard 2002). The concept of shell shock of the First World War was erroneous as it did not require shelling to be activated, nor was gross neurological shock or damage the cause of the disorder. Nevertheless, the First World War was associated with large numbers of soldiers being removed from the front line and some of them maintaining bizarre postures for days. Hysteria was frequently diagnosed.

Often sceptics suspect malingering – i.e. conscious feigning of dysfunction for tangible gain – in relation to hysterical presentations. This was frequently suspected to be the case in the First World War. Whether the immobile human wrecks removed from the front line should have been classed as suffering hysteria (nowadays known as conversion or dissociative disorders), PTSD, or more likely both – I cannot say. Both explanations may involve tonic immobility. However, even when staring death in the face, perception mediates the experience. Some may perceive their situation as hopeless, while others facing the same situation do not. The former may respond with tonic immobility while the latter fight and/or flee.

Further, if two equally brave soldiers were in the same immediate mortal danger, the more energy-depleted one would have a greater need for an energy-efficient defence – tonic immobility as opposed to fight or flight. The context of such First World War presentations was often of having experienced firepower and many other abominations on a scale never before experienced and for which troops had received inadequate preparation. Often they had suffered sleep deprivation and extended periods of living immersed in horror, death and futility. Some slept while standing in trenches pooled with water and woke later, finding their feet encased in ice. Often there was no realistic hope of survival (Shephard 2002). Perhaps tonic immobility was their last defence?

Hysterical neuroses are now far less common in western cultures than they were in the early twentieth century (Shorter 1986). While hysteria involves at times seemingly infantile psychological defences, it also is strongly associated with underlying organic disease.

I was referred a mature-age woman who came to my ward from a medical unit. She was behaving like a 4-year-old throwing an extended tearful tantrum. She appeared to have deliberate control of her actions. However, she also had a high pulse rate and fever, extremely high blood pressure and obvious neuro-logical signs. I returned her the same day to the medical unit whence she had come. From there she was admitted to inten-sive care, where she died ten days later of an astrocytoma (malignant brain tumour).

Hysteria is well known to psychiatrists as a potential trap for unwary medical personnel less familiar with it.

A recent detailed neuro-imaging investigation of a case of hyster-ical hemiparalysis of the left leg of two and a half years' duration found that the right anterior cingulate and right orbito-frontal cor-tex were responsible for inhibiting movement of the affected leg. The possibility of lack of effort was eliminated by the finding that when the unaffected leg was restrained and the subject prepared to move both legs, similar effects were found bilaterally in the motor areas responsible for movement preparation and execution (Marshall et al. 1997).

Kardiner (1941) suggested that sensorimotor disturbances (unable to feel or move) were the first combat stress symptoms to resolve, a notion that would be consistent with tonic immobility being an acute, transient and extreme defence. He also suggested there were three phases of the traumatic reaction: acute, transitional and stabilized, with the latter occurring after about two to three weeks. This is a timeframe within which only mental health workers working in war zones or disaster scenarios, or specializing in critical incident stress debriefing, would be familiar. Much of the PTSD seen in clinical practice has been established for many months or years. My clinical practice has many veterans with PTSD from the Vietnam War of the 1960s and a few from the Second World War, six decades after its end.

Future research directions

Tonic immobility being the last strategy of the defensive sequence differs greatly from attentive immobility, strongly suggesting different gene-neural mechanisms for the two forms of immobility. In lizards lesions of the striato-amygdaloid transition area (which is considered homologous with the mammalian central amygdala) reduce tonic immobility (Hueter et al. 2001). Cholinergic, opioid and gamma-aminobutyric acid (GABA) neurotransmission in the central amygdala have been found to inhibit tonic immobility in guinea pigs (Leite-Panissi and Menescal-de-Oliveira 2002). Also guinea pig research suggests that cholinergic stimulation of the lateral hypothalamus increases the duration of tonic immobility, while such stimulation of the medial and posterior hypothalamic regions modulates its duration (de Oliveira et al. 1997). There appears to be an interaction between opioid and cholinergic systems, with GABA inhibiting the duration of tonic immobility.

I have suggested that dissociation is probably a component of tonic immobility and vice versa. Might the study of tonic immobility yield objective clues to dissociation, one of the most puzzling of subjective experiences? Early research supports this suggestion. Under perceived threat, dissociative identity disorder (multiple personality) patients often become immobile, enter trance-like states and afterwards report out-of-body experiences, or dissociative amnesia (Nijenhuis et al. 1998). Further, the non-selective opioid receptor antagonist naltrexone has been found to reduce both dissociative phenomena and tonic immobility in patients with borderline personality disorder (which is related to PTSD) (Bohus et al.

1999). Sex differences in opioid-induced immobility have been found in rats stressed by foot shocks. Naloxone, another opioid antagonist, potentiated immobility in stressed males but not females (Klein et al. 1998). Might sex differences exist in humans? This possibility warrants investigation.

While the neural basis of tonic immobility is uncertain (Ramos et al. 1999), there are many data on the neurochemistry. Poultry have been extensively studied as they display this defence more prominently than most species and there is a considerable financial incentive to improve poultry management, including handling, as tonic immobility may affect the quality of the meat (e.g. Remignon et al. 1998). Serotonin agonists increase tonic immobility in chickens and serotonin antagonists do the reverse. Selective serotonin reuptake inhibitor drugs are used to treat PTSD. As they enhance serotonergic activity, this appears paradoxical. Chickens might respond differently from humans. Might such research be relevant to treatment of tonic immobility-related dissociation in humans?

Potential treatments worthy of exploration derived from poultry research are numerous, diverse, imaginative, bizarre and simple. Mostly, they are very long odds, but nothing ventured, nothing gained, and mostly they are very easy. They even include ascorbic acid (vitamin C). When ascorbic acid was administered to the drinking water of chickens for twenty-four hours prior to experimental handling, a decrease in the duration of tonic immobility was found (Zulkifli et al. 2000). However, other studies have not supported this. Similarly, cinanserin, a selective 5-HT2 antagonist has been found to reduce tonic immobility in birds.

An imaginative but bizarre example of exploring animal observations in humans is the idea of turning humans with dissociative problems partially, perhaps even totally, upside down (literally), using a modified 'tilt table'. It goes without saying that such an experiment would need meticulous ethical and safety measures approved by a research Ethics Committee. While not as sensitive as chickens or sharks to inversion, humans do have some tendency in this regard. If there is a link between tonic immobility and some forms of dissociation, those with relevant dissociative disorders or PTSD symptoms might demonstrate tonic immobility and/or its physiological indices upon inversion. The courts and genuine litigants might be delighted if this were so as it might serve as a test for malingering. However, I have little confidence in this particular idea. A small wager on an outsider is sometimes justified.

If this unlikely prospect happened to be confirmed, desensitization procedures might be conducted with inverted patients. Desensitization might start with simply being strapped onto a horizontal table with suitable reassurance and relaxation exercises. Thereafter, sessions might proceed with progressively increasing angles of tilt. In theory, extinction of the dissociative response might result.

> I recently discussed this bizarre experimental possibility with a patient with the rare dissociative identity disorder plus PTSD, with a history of extensive childhood sexual abuse. Coincidentally, she had been inverted on a tilt table at age 14 while undergoing a myelogram. She found it a terrifying experience. She was given minimal explanation of the procedure, was fully inverted (in one session) and received a painful injection into her spine. She also brought to my attention that during the years I have seen her, she has suffered periods lasting minutes of being unable to move while in dissociative states, which recently had decreased from monthly to once every few months. Her partner confirmed this. I was unaware of her immobility, as until then I had never asked.

My mention of vitamin C, cinanserin and experiments with inversion may all lead nowhere. However, my main message is who knows what else might be suggested by tapping unusual research sources. Poultry data are there to be examined by those with a little imagination.

> What is now proved was once only imagined.
> William Blake, 1757–1827

Conclusions

Tonic immobility represents the last defence available, when all preferable alternatives have become irrelevant. It is activated by situations involving proximity to, or touch by, the threat, restraint and overwhelming hopelessness. Rape and other civilian assaults involving these characteristics are contemporary contexts in which it may be activated. Tonic immobility also arises in war situations of overwhelming threat with no escape. The hysterical paralyses reported in the First and Second World Wars might have involved this mechanism and terminated sooner than symptoms reflecting other defensive mechanisms involved in PTSD. Nevertheless, scenarios reflecting the original trauma may reactivate it. One or more forms of dissociation may be the subjective counterparts of tonic immobility. If so, the extensive psychopharmacological data already available from animal research might help illuminate the neural substrate of dissociation.

Chapter 10

Agonic switching, preparedness and psychobiological response patterns

> False facts are highly injurious to the progress of science, for they often endure long; but false views, if supported by some evidence, do little harm, for everyone takes a salutary pleasure in proving their falseness.
>
> Charles Darwin, 1809–1882

Why do we not all suffer PTSD if it is adaptive?

Rachel Yehuda (1999) remarked, 'One of the critical problems in trying to understand the biology of PTSD is to address the issue of why only a proportion of trauma survivors develop a particular set of responses.' One part of the answer is likely to be genetic variance. Genetic research into psychiatric disorders is difficult at the best of times, but the requirement for research subjects to have suffered extraordinary stressors before family and twin studies can be undertaken, makes it even more so. PTSD is likely to involve multiple genes given the diversity of defences represented, learning, memory, preparedness and many other factors involved. Preliminary findings from twin studies strongly suggest heritability but these studies have not distinguished between genetic influences on trauma exposure versus that on PTSD as a reaction and type and severity of traumas have not been examined (Koenen 2003).

All evolutionary theories have as prerequisites gene-linked characteristics and inter-individual genetic variance. Without genetic variance there is no inheritance of variation and so no basis for evolution. Hence, from an evolutionary perspective 'genetic variance' is an unsatisfying answer for such an intriguing question. Nevertheless, it emphasizes the interactional nature of stressors impacting on organisms with specific genetic make-ups. Beyond genetic variance there has to be an activating mechanism or mechanisms for PTSD and its subthreshold manifestations. Furthermore, identical genomes can result in different phenotypes depending on environmental cues (Eisenberg 2004). Worker and queen bee larvae initially are identical, with differentiation arising from different feeding regimes.

Before we examine these mechanisms I must remind you that in Chapter 2, I stressed the importance of perception as a mediating variable (Foa and Kozac 1986; Yehuda and McFarlane 1995; McFarlane 1997). Remember, professional racing drivers emerge from horrific accidents without the frequency of PTSD associated with road traffic accidents. Hence, to the gene-neural variance answer, perception may be added. Further, from Chapter 3 we can suggest that important components of perception include predictability and controllability. Perception is also governed by the personality and life history of the individual. However, in this final chapter I wish to raise new issues pertinent to Yehuda's question.

If high-level defensive orientation has been adaptive, with PTSD being its extreme manifestation, why do we not routinely operate in this mode? Vigilance in animals carries the costs of decreased feeding and mating opportunities. It increases with increasing vulnerability to predators, decreasing certainty about predation risk, decreasing hunger and decreasing costs of lost opportunities (Sih 1990, 1992; Lima 1998). The irritability of PTSD is far from attractive to potential mates. As PTSD sufferers nowadays avoid supermarkets, so our distant ancestors would have limited their use of water holes and other exposure to predators. Our more recent ancestors would have been similarly influenced by conspecific risks.

The adaptiveness or maladaptiveness of PTSD is context dependent. Heightened defence is adaptive if the context is dangerous. The civilized times of today are times of plenty. This paradoxically increases vigilance in animals (Sih 1990, 1992). The relative safety of the present time is unlike the environments for which our genes evolved. I repeat the observation of primatologist, Craig Stanford (1998): 'Every wild primate dies after living a life of near-constant peril.'

Consider the following case from the perspective of survival in contemporary but less safe environments.

A coal miner developed the onset of panic attacks after finding that while working underground in a humid atmosphere, he had sustained extensive chemical burns. Subsequently, he was involved in an underground train crash in which he was flung into the end of a truck at 30–40 kph and feared he had broken his neck. More recently, explosives were prematurely activated only 50 metres from him. He was fortunate as he was partially protected from the blast and would have been killed if he had been checking these explosives. Subsequently, he became hypervigilant, unable to trust his colleagues and unreasonably checked their activities. Only weeks later he had a further accident, activating overt PTSD. An underground water/mudslide occurred, causing a machine to fall onto his ankle, trapping him for about one minute, during which time he was panic-stricken. He struggled to keep his head above water without hope of rescue, before the machine was swept off his leg, freeing him. His parents have encouraged him to quit mining. His PTSD is doing likewise.

Life in times of threat

The ancestral environment of primates, early hominids and contemporary hunter-gatherers involved much greater risks – than even of the present day's mining lifestyle. Nevertheless, many wild species operate much or most of the time in the 'hedonic mode'. This is a mood and behavioural state associated with affiliative social relations, mutual support and low arousal, which facilitates exploratory and creative behaviour (Chance 1988). The counterpart of the hedonic mode is the agonic mode. This is associated with high arousal, is conflict-orientated and according to Chance (1988) 'includes flight, withdrawal, freeze and submission, as well as elements of aggression.' Similarly, J.P. Scott writing in 1977 on human violence might have been writing about PTSD, when he wrote, 'The appropriate agonisitic behaviour may involve several alternatives: fight, flight, mutual avoidance, inactivity and so on.' The agonic mode is concerned with defence and is a system of behaviour that is adaptive in situations involving conflict. Dominance and submission characterize its relationships (Kudryavtseva 2000).

Both affiliative (hedonic) and competitive (agonic) behaviour in the right contexts reinforce social stability and group cohesion. The possibility that violence may in some contexts reinforce group cohesion may appear counterintuitive and offensive. Intuition is frequently a poor guide when it comes to evolution. Adolf Hitler's and Joseph Stalin's regimes were associated with high levels of national cohesion. An astute military commentator described to me observations consistent with this. Platoon leaders in times of war may gain respect from their troops from their preparedness to savagely enforce their dominance and control, even if at times their behaviour breaches military law. The same applies to criminally inclined motorcycle gangs.

The agonic switch

Even in the more hedonic species such as our own, threats may promote reciprocal agonic behaviour. In the agonic mode visual and spatial orientation reflect the constant consolidation and maintenance of the system. Subordinates stay within sight of the dominant individual and repeatedly gaze at him, making suitable adjustments in their behaviour. The dominant responds with suitably hostile or reassuring signals to maintain the required level of dominance/ subordination. Agonic subordinates have higher urinary output of adreno-corticosteroid hormones as seen in PTSD (Chance 1988).

Both hedonic and agonistic behaviours occur in wider social systems, which in turn are comprised of a number of subsystems (Scott 1977; Chance 1988). At the individual level the hypothalamo-pituitary adrenal axis regulates the output of stress hormones, which help orientate individuals to threats. At a social systems level, the same result occurs from a shift to agonistic interactions for threat reduction.

The onset of PTSD appears to be associated with an enduring switch from the hedonic to agonic mode. In ordinary hedonic life, rising anxiety improves performance for challenging tasks up to a certain anxiety level, beyond which performance efficiency declines. Life in war zones requires high arousal, vigilance and readiness to flee or attack according to contextual needs. From the perspective of PTSD these issues are relevant within the individual sufferers, their families, their closer social contacts and their broader social environments. Agonistic responses might be expected in all these subsystems.

The hedonic mode carries the benefits of social interaction and bonding but lacks the highly defensive vigilance of the agonic mode (Chance 1988). Conversely the agonic mode's defensive orientation is ill suited to bonding, socialization and exploration. Each strategy is associated with costs. The costs of the agonic switch are greater in hedonically orientated species such as ourselves, especially in civilized times. In an agonistically orientated species, becoming more defensive or aggressive may involve fewer costs. Two dogs savagely setting upon each other will get over the encounter much more quickly than if it had been their owners who had been in dispute.

Normally functioning social systems, even agonic ones, regulate violent behaviour, thereby reducing injuries. It is quite rare in nature and experimental situations to observe *strong* aggression because of multiple mechanisms inhibiting its manifestation (Kudryavtseva 2000). Aggression usually promotes polarization, whereby one individual becomes dominant and the other yields. Most conspecific violence is ritualistic – a display of machoism with little intent to seriously harm. This is referred to as ritualistic agonistic behaviour (Gilbert 1992). It represents a form of signalling behaviour as part of settling dominance subordination contests (Price 1988). The irritability of a PTSD sufferer reflects a heightened defensive orientation, signalling to the partner to behave in line with this.

Agonic and hedonic social systems may be represented in MacLean's (1949) concepts of reptilian, paleomammalian and neomammalian brain regions. Natalia Kudryavtseva (2000) from the Institute of Cytology and Genetics of the Siberian Division of the Russian Academy of Sciences has been exploring neurophysiological aspects of agonistic behaviour. Her work suggests an approach suitable for PTSD research, bridging the gap between a social systems and molecular research.

Kudryavtseva's (2000) experimental approach places the heaviest mice from different litters in experimental cages allowing them to see, hear and smell each other, but preventing physical contact. After two days 'eyeballing' each other, the barrier is removed and agonistic interactions ensue, establishing the victor and the vanquished. Victors then stay put in their cages (territory), but the vanquished are removed to unfamiliar cages with foreign-smelling litter, where they experience a series of manipulations involving encounters with other victors. Mice become repeatedly victorious or repeatedly defeated – a polarization of dominance and submissive orientations. The mice are then available for study of neurotransmitter changes reflecting agonistic polarity. Kudryavtseva (2000) claims this model corresponds well with and reflects psychogenic factors and events occurring in communities with unstable social processes and elevated levels of conflict.

Preparedness

Thus far we have the following answers as to why only some people develop PTSD when others experiencing similar traumas do not: genetic variance, perception (including predictability and controllability), context and the agonic switch. Can we take this further? In Chapter 3 I explained preparedness, which gives rise to rapid conditioning to fear and other survival stimuli, resistance to extinction and the easy reinstatement of extinguished symptoms characteristic of phobic states (Seligman 1971; Ohman and Mineka 2001).

Mammals modify defensive behaviours by adding to and reducing their innate fears by learning from direct or observed experiences with predators (Kavaliers and Choleris 2001), hostile conspecifics and threatening environments. Observational learning reduces the potential mortality associated with direct learning (Mineka and Cook 1986, 1993; Cook and Mineka 1987; Ohman 1986). Learning that snakes may be poisonous should not rely on personal experience. The more one reflects on snake-fear acquisition, the more essential observational and rapid learning appears. Snake fears represent an early evolutionary archetype.

Learning in relation to survival needs to be rapid and retained over time. If the response is potentially lifesaving, but infrequently required, it would be vulnerable to extinction. Preparedness meets the needs of rapid and enduring learning of survival responses (Cook and Mineka 1989; Ohman 1986). Being a primitive survival mechanism that evolved early, in the reptilian era if not earlier, we should not be surprised if it is insensitive to being switched off. It is better to be safe than sorry. The agonic switch fulfils the need for the adjustment of defensive mode; preparedness facilitates this switch.

Preparedness must be at least partially genetically determined. Regrettably, most psychiatric genetic research has used disease models. Tsuang and colleagues (2004) have emphasized the need for research to recognize interactive effects between genes and environmental contexts, with different environments providing different opportunities for genetic potentials to be actualized.

Non-archetypal traumas

Snakes, predators, fires and many other life-threatening traumas involve brain archetypes handed down over ancestral time, by way of genetically facilitated learning mechanisms. Our ancestors did not drive motor vehicles and so there can be no specific genetic representation of them. Yet, transport accidents do activate PTSD. Again, might the theory break down? I suggest not. Such accidents may activate archetypal fears associated with predation and other ancestral traumas. A Second World War pilot, who suffers PTSD, illustrates this.

> Mr X was an exceptional fighter pilot. One day, running low on fuel, he had to switch to the reserve fuel tank. There was a problem with the switch-over mechanism and he could not access the spare tank. Shortly afterwards he ran out of fuel. His plane was one that 'glided like a brick' and so he had to put it into a steep dive to maintain control. He fortunately found a field and successfully landed the plane, but it ploughed through a wire fence. When it came to a halt he was trapped, as the wire had wrapped itself around the canopy. After ten minutes of extreme fear of being incinerated, he successfully escaped.
>
> As is often the case with PTSD, Mr X suffered a number of traumas. Subsequently, he was a passenger being flown in a small plane by a pilot who 'obviously could not fly'. Mr X was in no doubt that his life was in serious danger. A few days later the incompetent pilot fatally crashed. A third trauma occurred when Mr X was on airfield duty. A single-propeller aircraft landed and swerved out of control into a crowd of bystanders. Limbs severed by the propeller flew everywhere. Mr X is haunted by a particular image of a body that was hurled into the treetops and bounced from branch to branch as it fell to the ground.

Mr X's first two experiences involved fears associated with falling from a great height and then entrapment. Entrapment is usually fatal if a predator is involved and often so when a conspecific or the environment are the villains. The third incident involved limbs torn from bodies, as in some sort of predatory nightmare. Hence, the genetically sterile technology of modern transport may recreate entrapment or carnage similar to that of predation or other archetypes, which are reflected in our genes.

Psychobiological response patterns

While conditioning psychology has described preparedness, evolutionary psychology uses the overlapping concepts of 'psychobiological response patterns' (Gilbert 1992) and 'response rules' (Wenegrat 1984). In a defence context, response rules dictate that serious threats will activate specific context-dependent defensive psychobiological responses. These include all the defences that I have discussed. However, there is a subtle difference in emphasis. 'Defence' implies just defence. 'Response rules' imply 'if A is occurring in situation B, then C is the correct response'. Psychobiological response patterns are behavioural responses to specific biologically recurring circumstances and are governed by response rules. Appeasement is an example of a psychobiological response pattern, involving a hedonic strategy under agonic circumstances involving a dominant conspecific aggressor (or aggressors) and entrapment. Much of its adaptiveness lies in its potential to stimulate a hedonic switch in the aggressor.

The 'apprehension continuum' concept involves a range of vigilant behaviours by prey in response to perceived predation risk (Kavaliers and Choleris 2001). Response rules dictate that vigilance will be adjusted according to perceived risk, but the costs of so doing have to be carefully balanced in a trade-off. Prey animals can decrease their activity and use different temporal (day or night) and spatial refuges to reduce their vulnerability. Some prey are exposed to chronic risk, others more sporadic. Prey that infrequently encounter predators can afford a greater pulse of reduced activity – going without food occasionally is a more acceptable cost for cautious behaviour than going without food regularly (Miller 2002).

What are the implications of this for present-day civilization? The low hazard existence of developed nations nowadays would favour a more extreme response to acute hazards. Those of the most disadvantaged nations (and in ancestral times) might starve if they responded similarly to their more frequent hazards. From an evolutionary perspective energy-depleted individuals, those starving or pregnant, need to take greater risks to survive than those more replete (Lima and Dill 1990; Lima 1998).

In PTSD the experienced traumas are often outside the usual range of experiences for which individuals are prepared. Under circumstances where customary defensive behaviour is proving, or has proved, seriously deficient a higher order of response rules is selected. Preparedness in this context will facilitate the activation of innate psychobiological defensive responses that have been held in reserve, the extreme end of which we know as PTSD.

While agonic exchanges may activate psychobiological response patterns based on fear, they may also activate responses we know as 'depression' – a particularly vague term spanning a range of cognitions including loss, shame, guilt, hopelessness and others, all of which have specific evolutionary functions. Conspecific-induced traumas such as rape and other assaults induce not only defensive behaviour but also loss of status. Involuntary subordinate status involves feeling put down and kept down (Price 1988; Gilbert 1992). This status loss form of depression evolved as a yielding subroutine of ritual agonistic behaviour (Price and Sloman 1987) and according to the evolutionary theory might be expected to frequently complicate conspecific-induced PTSD. Status loss can also arise from environmental and predator-related traumas indirectly by way of loss of functional capacity. These different phenomena will be associated with different neuroanatomical and neurochemical systems. The fact that trauma will often activate both fear- and loss-based modules does not negate the importance of considering them as separate entities.

Trauma contexts and responses

The traditional psychopathological model of PTSD tends to suggest one severe trauma-related illness resulting from diverse severe traumas. Van Praag (2004) has suggested that the diffuse concept of stress is an obstacle to progress. Stress is too heterogeneous for biological research. Different physiological responses may be expected from different psychological phenomena. The evolutionary model proposed suggests that the concept of PTSD should be reserved for fear-related reactions. Furthermore, the theory proposes that fear is merely the emotional response serving vigilance and the various defensive responses. The latter will be selected according to context. Contextual elements include the nature of the trauma (being attacked, being caught in a fire, etc.), who or what inflicted it, their motivation (if applicable), the environment (trauma in one's home suggests nowhere is safe), the prior life history of individuals experiencing the traumas and the ensuing consequences.

While specific context-dependent defensive reactions will be activated under normal circumstances, this may not be so in those experiencing abnormally severe and sustained traumatic reactions. Nevertheless, consideration should be given to the possibility that particular traumas, in specific contexts, may induce specific and therefore predictable traumatic responses as suggested by the concepts of response rules and psychobiological response patterns. Consideration of these reactions should be based on vigilance and the six key mammalian defences.

Research to date has neglected such considerations, but there is some evidence suggesting specific reactions. I have already reviewed the six key defences. In addition, data that have not been based on these defences have suggested some specific reactions. Rape victims attacked in their beds tend to experience fear of being at home, whereas those attacked outside their homes experience the reverse (Burgess and Holmstrom 1974). Being raped in an extremely dangerous part of town, traumatic though it may be, might allow a woman the security of knowing that in other parts of town, the risk is less. Further, the sense of betrayal by fellow man may be less.

Victims of single traumas such as assaults and disasters display fewer numbing symptoms than those with repeated traumas, and the former have also been found to experience disproportionately high rates of re-experiencing symptoms compared with other symptoms (cited by Foa et al. 1992). The evolutionary theory predicts this, as a single trauma would be easier to forget than a series of traumas. The painful repeated re-experiencing of a single trauma reminds the individual not to revert to unwary habits. The National Vietnam Readjustment Study (US) found that while re-experiencing symptoms declined over a two-year period, avoidance symptoms increased (Kulka et al. 1990), again consistent with the proposed evolutionary theory. If avoidance is more reliable, reminders are less necessary. PTSD changes with time and may involve a series of transitional states (McFarlane 1997). However, the mechanisms underlying these transitional states remain unclear.

In contrast, with repeated traumas there is more need to prevent becoming psychologically overwhelmed. Numbing symptoms are more prevalent in victims of repeated abuse (Foa et al. 1992). We have also seen that excessive appeasement is a trauma response specific to protracted abusive control (Herman 1992) by a dominant conspecific and that some types of dissociation may be related to tonic immobility, which is also highly context dependent.

Analgesia is of obvious adaptive value in a flight or fight situation. Hence, it is to be expected that numbing might be prominent early in the course of PTSD and there is at least some evidence that this may be so (Scurfield 1985), although further research is needed. Whether non-analgesic forms of numbing might be prominent early in the course also warrants consideration.

High levels of intrusive (re-experiencing) symptoms have been found in combat veterans (Laufer et al. 1985; True et al. 1993). Soldiers, who may later develop PTSD, generally have been required to ignore their avoidant instincts until they were released from their combat obligations. It would not be incompatible with the theory if nature inflicted memory lessons (re-experiencing symptoms) on such individuals who appear to have ignored its message for so long.

I have volunteered these few selected observations on symptom profiles suggesting PTSD responses may be specific to their contexts. However, much more definitive work is needed using uniform methodology to isolate which symptoms arise, with what frequencies, in which situations. The neurobiology is likely to be different not only for re-experiencing, avoidance and overarousal/hypervigilance categories, but also for many of the symptoms within. Split-second startle phenomena are very different from protracted hypervigilance/wariness. Further, the startle reflex is reptilian in origin, whereas the signalling function of irritability suggests more recent mammalian contributions.

Davis and Whalen (2001) have asserted that their neuroscientific studies suggest that anxiety disorders might be better understood as disorders of vigilance. The more ecological evolutionary perspective developed in this book concurs with this suggestion. If PTSD is adaptive it involves fear requiring a specific response to the context in which it occurs. There are discrete gene-neural modules of responses waiting to be activated and these psychobiological responses are subject to cost–benefit considerations similar to 'prey decision-making'. PTSDs (plural) might be better conceptualized as disorders of vigilance and risk assessment, combined with the six defensive strategies and utilized according to contextual determinants including cost–benefit considerations.

Conclusions

Peaceful existence is associated with the hedonic mode. Threats activate agonistic behaviour. All humans have this potential awaiting activation, producing mostly short-term responses. The stressors that may activate PTSD disturb virtually all persons, as demonstrated in studies of disaster victims with subthreshold PTSD symptomatology. PTSD represents an unusually severe and persistent agonic activation. A number of species-specific behaviours are represented in gene-neural brain circuitry, but require activation. Such activation involves 'preparedness'. Preparedness provides for rapid learning, often from a single exposure producing enduring results and is the mechanism underlying agonic switching. Persistent agonic behaviour involves costs. However, if the context appears sufficiently threatening, a switch to habitual agonistic orientation may have been adaptive in ancestral times. Consideration of trauma must involve cost–benefit equations associated with specific contexts and responses to them. There is preliminary evidence suggesting that some symptoms of PTSD may be context specific. PTSD may be viewed as a psychobiological response pattern activated by the perception of archetypal fears associated with prey decision-making.

Putting this all together with the defensive nature of PTSD suggested from Chapters 5–9, we have the following: PTSD may be conceptualized as a disorder of vigilance and risk assessment, combined with the six mammalian defences, activated according to contextual determinants, including perception (influenced by gene-neural variance, life histories, predictability, controllability and other factors) and cost–benefit considerations. The mechanism of action involves further gene-neural variance, preparedness and psychobiological response patterns employed according to context-dependent response rules and results in an enduring shift from the hedonic to agonic mode. Given the number of variables involved, great variability in traumatic reactions would be expected. This goes some way to answering the fascinating question of why trauma causes only a proportion of a population to develop PTSD.

> God could cause us considerable embarrassment by revealing all the secrets of nature to us: we should not know what to do for sheer apathy and boredom.
>
> J. W. von Goethe, 1749–1832

PTSD in other species?

> Mankind differs from the animals only by a little, and most people throw that away.
>
> Confucius, c. 551–479 BC

PTSD may well exist in many species, although this remains to be demonstrated. If this turns out to be the case, we have much to learn by studying the phenomenon in animals, preferably in their natural environments for which their defences evolved. It amazed me in the earlier stages of this work that so little research has been conducted on the long-term outcome of prey animals surviving near misses with predators. Numerous inquiries of key contacts and institutions, and the networks that flowed from these, revealed little other than that animal behaviourists suspect that PTSD does exist – in pets at least.

Animals suffering PTSD would stand out as unusually avoidant, hypervigilant (both regarding watchfulness and physiological hyper-arousal) and prone to unusually aggressive responses in a generalized way. Re-experiencing phenomena may be more subjective than avoidance and overarousal symptoms, but even pets can be observed to experience them; for example, a traumatized dog may whine or howl when reminded of the trauma and attack if approached by a stranger. Maltreated pets, such as dogs and cats, are known to display these key overly defensive phenomena.

Veterinary practice lends itself well to PTSD research. Vast numbers of dogs and cats are taken to veterinary surgeries having been run over by motor vehicles and a minority might be expected to develop PTSD, if it exists in those species.

Some years ago, my own Burmese cat returned home one day, with a gashed head and covered in oil. Presumably it had gone under a moving vehicle. For two years afterwards, I observed that if it was in our quiet front garden and a vehicle passed by, it would flee into the house in obvious alarm. My reaction was, 'Good. That will increase her chances of survival.' An unsympathetic attitude perhaps, but evolution does not care at all. The cat did not display generalization of anxiety nor become aggressive, so I do not suggest it had full PTSD. However, it did appear to have subthreshold symptoms. A few years following its seemingly complete recovery, we moved to a temporary home next to a busy road. In our three months there the cat became markedly reclusive, preferring a particular bedroom and became uncharacteristically overweight. Our second Burmese cat coped with this temporary home without behavioural change. The first one quickly returned to a happier state and shed its excess weight when we moved to our final home away from traffic.

These observations may be coincidental, but are not inconsistent with what might be expected for mild PTSD reactivation by proximity to traffic, the source of the original trauma.

The diagnosis of PTSD should be reserved for generalized avoidance and flight responses. A dog that has been run over and develops PTSD would be more generally avoidant and hypervigilant, perhaps with exaggerated startle and other fear responses such as cowering. Most importantly for veterinary practice, it may also be uncharacteristically prone to aggressive defence – i.e. it might be snappy – making it a liability and increasing the probability of it being brought to a vet's attention.

If approximately 15 per cent of human motor vehicle casualties develop PTSD, might a similar proportion of pets in not too dissimilar circumstances also do so? I have suggested that the hedonic lifestyle of *Homo sapiens*, especially during civilization, may promote higher rates of PTSD than might be found in more natural and more agonic environments. Pets exist in civilization, but retain more of their wild instincts than do the so-called wisest of the great apes. Accordingly, I would expect rates of PTSD in pets to be intermediate between those of modern humans and contemporary wildlife.

Chronic human maltreatment of pets might instil a relationship of appeasement crossing species. For example, a dog may loyally support its cruel owner. As humans are not kept captive by other species, appeasement in humans is limited to conspecifics. This may not be the case in animals, though different animal species might behave differently in this regard.

While veterinary research provides for simple research designs that would be within reach of most vets having access to research resources, observations of non-domesticated animals in their natural environments might provide the ultimate revelations. Naturalistic and ecological studies would be more costly to conduct, but correspondingly more illuminating. How does a young wildebeest that has survived a mauling by a large predator respond? Perhaps quite unremarkably. Most humans do not develop PTSD following traumas. Therefore *populations* of traumatized animals would need to be studied, as only a minority would be expected to develop PTSD. Further, I have suggested that humans and therefore non-humans living in states of frequent threat may be less vulnerable to such threats – as if they had been inoculated against stress according to behaviourist terminology. The evolutionary theory supported by sound research suggests that the costs of widespread avoidance of predators might simply be too great in the relevant environments (Lima 1998; Miller 2002).

The ideal trauma to study in the wild would be an 'unpredicted' one generating a sense of 'uncontrollability', as we know from laboratory studies on animals and human research that these factors are powerful inducers of fear and long-term anxiety. In many developed nations forest fires may provide a suitable traumatic arena for such studies. Forest fires inflict massive trauma on many animals that are unable to find shelter, e.g. by retreating underground. Regrettably, even the rainforests in South East Asia have recently provided such disaster scenarios for non-human primates including the orangutan. It would in theory be possible to examine diverse species' responses to such traumas with no shortage of numbers, rare species excepted. The challenge would be the future tracking of individuals to assess outcomes. Follow-up periods would need to be a minimum of three months or so. The use of transmitters might facilitate such exercises. The rescue and rehabilitation of severely injured animals might provide easier opportunity for observations, but carry the disadvantage of the additional trauma of being removed from their natural environments. However, if they have already been captured for rehabilitation, releasing them with tracking devices for assessment of outcomes is clearly feasible given sufficient resources.

The ultimate studies of non-domesticated animals in their natural environments might be studies of primates, especially chimpanzees and bonobos, because of their genetic and social similarities to humans. I would predict that the gentler bobobo might have a lower threshold for traumatization than the more violent chimpanzee. In our own species, males are exposed to more traumatic events, but females are more likely to develop PTSD given a particular trauma. Both chimpanzees and bonobos are vulnerable to predators but perhaps not as routinely as are many other primates and other non-primate species. Chimpanzees also have an additional research attribute, namely their inclination to kill their own species as we do ourselves. Hence, chimpanzees may provide naturalistic observations with respect to both predator and conspecific-induced traumas. Their close relationships to ourselves suggests that if any non-human species suffer PTSD, then chimpanzees and bonobos should do so.

Glossary

Adaptive conservatism A tendency for successful evolutionary attributes to be preserved across evolutionary time.

Adrenocorticotrophic hormone (ACTH) is released from the anterior pituitary gland, leading to the release of glucocorticoids from the adrenal gland.

Agonic mode A type of interaction characterized by competition for status resolved by a dominant subordinate polarity.

Algorithms Genetically mediated mechanisms resulting in patterns of functional behaviours, analogous to Jung's 'archetypes'.

Amygdala A key limbic brain structure responsible for the evaluation of the emotional meaning of incoming stimuli, e.g. fear.

Ancestral environment The environment for which our genes evolved.

Appeasement Pacification/conciliation, defence strategy used by a subordinate to a dominant.

Atrophy Wasting due to disease or lack of use.

Australopithecines The earlier ancestors of *Homo* emerging from the common ancestor of humans, chimpanzees and bonobos.

Basal ganglia Brain nuclei that regulate movement; the 'reptilian' part of the brain serving essential bodily functions.

Classical conditioning Associative learning involving pairing of a neutral stimulus (conditioned stimulus) with a stimulus (unconditioned) that produces a result (conditioned response) without need for learning.

Coevolution The simultaneous interactive evolution of two or more species.

Comorbidity The co-occurrence of two or more psychiatric disorders in one person.

Complex PTSD PTSD in which the subsequent developmental course of the individual is disrupted – usually due to trauma in childhood.

Conditioned stimulus/response   The associative learning of a new stimulus/response following pairing with unconditioned stimuli/responses, e.g. pain/fear.

Conservatism   Tendency for evolved attributes to persist over long periods, often because of the non-viability of genetic leaps.

Conspecific   A member of the same species.

Convergence   Two species resembling each other because of shared environmental evolutionary challenge, as opposed to genetic similarity.

Cortex   More recently developed region of the brain responsible for higher cognitive functions.

Corticotrophin releasing factor (CRF)   A neuropeptide secreted by the hypothalamus triggering release of adrenocorticotrophic hormone from the pituitary gland and thereby activating the stress response.

Crypsis   Morphological or behavioural attributes that facilitate an animal remaining undetected.

***Diagnostic and Statistical Manual of Mental Disorders* (DSM)**   Influential American classificatory scheme.

Dissociation   A split between the 'observing self' and the 'experiencing self'.

Dissociative identity disorder (DID)   Formerly multiple personality disorder.

Dominant   A conspecific of leading status.

Evolutionarily stable strategy   A mathematical conceptualization of evolutionary strategies. Stable strategies cannot be outperformed by alternative strategies in the long term.

Extinction   Reduction in learnt response due to withdrawal or lack of reinforcement.

Eye movement desensitization and reprocessing (EMDR)   A behavioural treatment used for PTSD.

Fitness   Relative reproductive success.

Gamma-aminobutyric acid (GABA)   An inhibitory brain neurotransmitter.

Genotype   The genetic make-up of an individual.

Habituation   A form of learning involving reduction in response over time – involving growing accustomed to the potential threat.

Hedonic mode   Affiliative relationships involving cooperation and facilitation of exploratory behaviour.

Hippocampus   Closely related to the amygdala, it records in memory the spatial and time-related aspects of emotional experience.

Hominids   Upright bipedal apes.

Hypothalamo-pituitary adrenal axis   A stress response system involving the hypothalamus, pituitary and adrenal glands.

Hypothalamus   Part of the brain playing a key role in the integration of autonomic and endocrine functions, intimately related to the pituitary gland and connecting with the limbic system and cortex.

Inclusive fitness   The genetic survival potential including descendants carrying the individual's genes.

In-group   Conspecifics accepting each other.

Interspecific   Between species.

Intraspecific   Within a species.

Limbic system   An ill-defined system responsible for emotions; the 'paleomammalian' brain.

Natural selection   The tendency for survival over evolutionary time of genes (and individuals) with advantageous characteristics.

Neocortex   'New brain'; more recently developed brain with cognitive functions.

Neomammalian   The era of the development of the neocortex ('neocortical' and 'neomammalian' are synonyms).

Neurogenesis   The production of neurons.

Operant conditioning   Behavioural learning influenced by rewards and punishments.

Out-group   Conspecifics not accepted by the main (in-)group.

Paleomammalian   The earlier mammalian era.

Phenomenology   Understanding of mental disorders based on what is observed as opposed to theoretical understanding.

Phylogeny   The evolutionary origin and development of species.

Plasticity   Change in neuronal connectivity in proportion to experience ('use it or lose it').

Posttraumatic stress disorder (PTSD)   A psychological disorder affecting individuals who have experienced or witnessed profoundly traumatic events, such as torture, murder, rape or wartime combat, characterized by recurrent flashbacks of the traumatic event, nightmares, irritability, anxiety, fatigue, forgetfulness and social withdrawal.

Prefrontal cortex   Area of the cortex behind the forehead; the location of self-will.

Preparedness   Learning facilitated by its relevance to evolutionary necessities.

Primates   Monkeys, lemurs and apes.

Psychobiological response pattern   A predetermined behavioural response to some biologically recurring circumstance.

Psychoneural   A word implying unity of psychological and neurological.

Punctuated equilibrium   A period of stasis or little change followed by rapid change, in a lineage.

Reciprocal altruism   Evolutionary term referring to helping non-kin on a 'you scratch my back and I'll scratch yours' basis.

Reptilian brain   The most primitive aspect of the triune brain with substantially reflex actions.

Resource holding potential   Capacity for fighting; extent of resources; power basis.

Response rules   The basis on which psychobiological response patterns may operate. It is context dependent.

Reverted escape   Return of a defeated/subordinate individual to the dominant (in contrast to flight).

Ritual agonistic behaviour   A characteristic power display or signalling with relative restraint from violence.

Selection   Mechanism of evolutionary change based on advantageous characteristics, which over time will be selected for by reproductively outperforming alternative characteristics.

Selective serotonin reuptake inhibitors (SSRIs)   A group of antidepressants.

Sociobiology   Behavioural study based on the survival of genes ultimately driving behavioural characteristics.

Subcortical   Brain region or functioning other than neocortical; reptilian and paleomammalian regions and functions outside of conscious awareness.

Subordinate   A conspecific of lesser status.

Thalamus   A major relay station for incoming information to brain areas.

Triune brain   Concept introduced by Paul McLean; involves reptilian, paleomammalian and neomammalian regions and functions.

Unconditioned stimulus/response   A stimulus producing a specific response without need for learning.

References

Aarts, P.G.H. and Op den Velde, W. (1996) Prior traumatization and the process of aging: theory and clinical implications. In: *Traumatic Stress: the effects of overwhelming experience on mind, body, and society*. Eds: van der Kolk, B.A., McFarlane, A.C. and Weisaeth, L. New York: Guilford.

Ahern, J., Galea, S., Resnick, H., Kilpatrick, D., Bucuvalas, M., Gold, J. and Vlahov, D. (2002) Television images and psychological symptoms after September 11 terrorist attacks. *Psychiatry*, 65: 289–300.

Albeck, D., McKittrick, C., Blanchard, R., Nikulina, J., McEwen, B. and Sakai, R. (1997) Chronic social stress alters levels of corticotrophin-releasing factor and arginine vasopressin mRNA in rat brain. *Neuroscience*, 17: 4895–4903.

Alberts, S.C. (1994) Vigilance in young baboons: effects of habitat, age, sex and maternal rank on glance rate. *Animal Behaviour*, 47: 749–755.

Alexander, R.D. (1979) *Darwinism and Human Affairs*. Seattle, WA: University of Washington Press.

Anisman, H. (1978) Neurochemical changes elicited by stress: behavioural correlates. In: *Psychopharmacology of Aversively Motivated Behavior*. Eds: Anisman, H. and Bignami, G. New York: Plenum Press.

APA (1980) *Diagnostic and Statistical Manual of Mental Disorders*, 3rd edn. Washington, DC: American Psychiatric Association.

APA (1994) *Diagnostic and Statistical Manual of Mental Disorders*, 4th edn. Washington, DC: American Psychiatric Association.

APA (2000) *Diagnostic and Statistical Manual of Mental Disorders*, 4th edn, revised. Washington, DC: American Psychiatric Association.

Artwohl, A. and Christensen, L.W. (1997) *Deadly Force Encounters*. Boulder, CO: Paladin Press.

Auerbach, S.M., Kiesler, D.J., Strentz, T., Schmidt, J.A. and Devany Serio, C. (1994) Interpersonal impacts and adjustment to the stress of simulated captivity: an empirical test of the Stockholm syndrome. *Journal of Social and Clinical Psychology*, 2: 207–221.

Bargh, J.A. and Chartrand, T.L. (1999) The unbearable automaticity of being. *American Psychologist*, 54: 462–479.

Basoglu, M. and Mineka, S. (1992) The role of uncontrollable and unpredictable stress in posttraumatic stress responses in torture survivors. In: *Torture and its Consequences: current treatment approaches.* Ed: Basoglu, M. Cambridge: Cambridge University Press.

Beahrs, J.O. (1990) The evolution of posttraumatic behavior: three hypotheses. *Dissociation Progress in the Dissociative Disorders,* 31: 15–21.

Beveridge, A. (1997) On the origins of posttraumatic stress disorder. In: *Psychological Trauma: a developmental approach.* Eds: Black, D., Newman, M., Harris-Hendriks, J. and Mezey, G. London: Gaskell.

Birx, H.J. (1997) Introduction. In: *The Descent of Man,* by Charles Darwin. Loughton, UK: Prometheus.

Bisson, J. (2003) Ministry of Defense war trauma case discussed in plenary session, ECOTS Berlin. *Traumatic Stress Points,* 17: 7.

Blanchard, D.C., Blanchard, R.J. and Rodgers, J. (1991) Risk assessment and animal models of anxiety. In: *Animal Models in Psychopharmacology.* Eds: Olivier, B., Mos, J. and Slangen, J.L. Basel: Birkhauser Verlag AG.

Blanchard, R.J., Yudko, E.B., Rodgers, R.J. and Blanchard, D.C. (1993) Defense system psychopharmacology: an ethological approach to the pharmacology of fear and anxiety. *Behavioural Brain Research,* 58: 155–165.

Blanchard, R.J., Nikulina, J.N., Sakai, R.R., McKittrick, C., McEwen, B. and Blanchard, C. (1998) Behavior and endocrine change following chronic predatory stress. *Physiology and Behavior,* 63: 561–569.

Boesch, C. (1991) The effects of leopard predation on grouping patterns in forest chimpanzees. *Behaviour,* 117: 220–242.

Bohus, M.J., Landwehrmeyer, G.B., Stiglmayr, C.E., Limberger, M.F., Bohme, R. and Schmahl, C.G. (1999) Naltrexone in the treatment of dissociative symptoms in patients with borderline personality disorder: an open label trial. *Journal of Clinical Psychiatry,* 60: 598–603.

Bolles, R.C. (1970) Species-specific defense reactions and avoidance learning. *Psychological Review,* 77: 32–48.

Bourne, P.B., Rose, R.M. and Mason, J.W. (1968) 17-OHCS levels in combat: special forces 'A' team under threat of attack. *Archives of General Psychiatry* 19: 135–140.

Bremner, J.D., Southwick, S.M. and Charney, D.S. (1999) The neurobiology of posttraumatic stress disorder: an integration of animal and human research. In: *Posttraumatic Stress Disorder: a comprehensive text.* Eds: Saigh, P.A. and Bremner, J.D. Needham Heights, MA: Allyn and Bacon.

Breslau, N., Kessler, R.C., Chilcoat, H.D., Schultz, L.R., Davis, G.C. and Andreski, P. (1998) Trauma and posttraumatic stress disorder in the community: the 1996 Detroit Area Survey of Trauma. *Archives of General Psychiatry,* 55: 626–632.

Breslau, N., Cilcoat, H.D., Kessler, R.C., Peterson, E.L. and Lucia, V.C. (1999) Vulnerability to assaultive violence: further specification of the sex difference in posttraumatic stress disorder. *Psychological Medicine*, 29: 813–821.

Brett, E.A. (1996) The classification of posttraumatic stress disorder. In: *Traumatic Stress: the effects of overwhelming experience on mind, body, and society*. Eds: van der Kolk, B.A., McFarlane, A.C. and Weisaeth, L. New York: Guilford.

Brodie, E.D. Jr, Formanowicz, D.R. Jr and Brodie, E.D. III (1991) Predator avoidance and antipredator mechanisms: distinct pathways to survival. *Ethology Ecology and Evolution*, 3: 73–77.

Bryant, R.A. and Harvey, A.G. (2002) Delayed-onset posttraumatic stress disorder: a prospective evaluation. *Australian and New Zealand Journal of Psychiatry*, 36: 205–209.

Burgess, A.W. and Holmstrom, L.L. (1974) *American Journal of Psychiatry*, 131: 981–986.

Buss, D.M. (1991) Evolutionary personality psychology. *Annual Reviews in Psychology*, 42: 459–491.

Carter, R. (1998) *Mapping the Mind*. London: Phoenix.

Chance, M.R.A. (1988) *Social Fabrics of the Mind*. Hove: Lawrence Erlbaum.

Chapman, C.A., Wrangham, R.W. and Chapman, L.J. (1995) Ecological constraints on group size: an analysis of spider monkey and chimpanzee subgroups. *Behavioural Ecology and Sociobiology*, 36: 59–70.

Chemtob, C., Roitblat, H.C., Ramada, R.S., Carlson, J.G. and Twentyman, C.T. (1988) A cognitive action theory of posttraumatic stress disorder. *Journal of Anxiety Disorders*, 2: 253–275.

Chemtob, C.H., Tolin, D.F., van der Kolk, B.A. and Pitman, R.K. (2000) Eye movement desensitization and reprocessing (Chapters 7 and 19). In: *Effective Treatments for PTSD*. Eds: Foa, E.B., Keane, T.M. and Friedman, M.J. New York: Guilford.

Cook, M. and Mineka, S. (1987) Second-order conditioning and over-shadowing in the observational conditioning of fear in monkeys. *Behavior Research and Therapy*, 25: 349–364.

Cook, M. and Mineka, S. (1989) Observational conditioning of fear to fear-relevant versus fear-irrelevant stimuli in rhesus monkeys. *Journal of Abnormal Psychology*, 98: 448–459.

Coplan, J., Trost, R., Owens, M., Cooper, T., Gorman, J., Nemeroff, C. and Rosenbaum, L. (1998) Cerebrospinal fluid concentrations of somatostatin and biogenic amines in grown primates reared by mothers exposed to manipulated foraging conditions. *Archives of General Psychiatry*, 55: 473–477.

Crowley, P.H., Travers, S.E., Linton, M.C., Cohn, S.L., Sih, A. and Sargent, R.C. (1991) Male density, predation risk, and the seasonal sequence of mate choices: a dynamic game. *American Naturalist*, 137: 567–596.

Curio, E. (1988) Cultural transmission of enemy recognition by birds. In:

Social Learning: psychological and biological perspectives. Eds: Zentall, T.R. and Galef, B.G. Hillsdale, NJ: Lawrence Erlbaum.

Daly, M. and Wilson, M. (1988) *Homicide*. New York: Aldine de Gruyter.

Daly, R.J. (1983) Samuel Pepys and posttraumatic stress disorder. *British Journal of Psychiatry*, 143: 64–68.

Darwin, C. (1871) *The Descent of Man* (2003 edn). London: Gibson Square Books.

Davidson, J.R.T. and van der Kolk, B.A. (1996) The psychopharmacological treatment of posttraumatic stress disorder. In: *Traumatic Stress: the effects of overwhelming experience on mind, body, and society*. Eds: van der Kolk, B.A., McFarlane, A.C. and Weisaeth, L. New York: Guilford.

Davis, M. and Whalen, P.J. (2001) The amygdala: vigilance and emotion. *Molecular Psychiatry*, 6: 13–34.

Dawkins, R. (1976) *The Selfish Gene*. Oxford: Oxford University Press.

Deahl, M. (2000) Psychological debriefing: controversy and challenge. *Australian and New Zealand Journal of Psychiatry*, 34: 929–939.

De Bellis, M. (2001) Developmental traumatology: the psychobiological development of maltreated children and its implications for research, treatment, and policy. *Development and Psychopathology*, 13: 539–564.

De Oliveira, L., Hoffmann, A. and Menescal-de-Oliveira, L. (1997) The lateral hypothalamus in the modulation of tonic immobility in guinea pigs. *Neuroreport*, 8: 3489–3493.

De Waal, F.B.M. (1988) The reconciled hierarchy. In: *Social Fabrics of the Mind*. Ed: Chance, M.R.A. Hove: Lawrence Erlbaum.

Dixon, A.K. (1998) Ethological strategies for defence in animals and humans: their role in some psychiatric disorders. *British Journal of Medical Psychology*, 71: 417–455.

Dodman, N.H. and Shuster, L. (1998) *Psychopharmacology of Animal Behavior Disorders*. Malden, MA: Blackwell Science.

Dunbar, R.I.M. (1996) *Grooming, Gossip and the Evolution of Language*. Cambridge, MA: Harvard University Press.

Edlund, B. (1995–1996) *Homo Erectus*. Origins of Human Kind Research Center. http://www.pro-am.com/origins/research/erectus1.htm

Egendorf, A., Kadushin, C., Laufer, R.S., Rothbart, G. and Sloan, L. (1981) *Legacies of Veterans and their Peers*. New York: Center for Policy Research.

Eisenberg, L. (2004) Social psychiatry and the human genome: contextualizing heritability. *British Journal of Psychiatry*, 184: 101–103.

Ember, C.R. (1978) Myths about hunter-gatherers. *Ethnology*, 17: 439–448.

Endler, J.A. (1986) Defence against predators. In: *Predator–Prey Relationships: perspectives and approaches from the study of lower vertebrates*. Eds: Feder, M.E. and Lauder, G.V. Chicago, IL, and London: University of Chicago Press.

Eriksson, P.S., Perfilieva, E., Bjork-Eriksson, T., Alborn, A., Nordborg, C.,

Peterson, D.A. and Gage, F.H. (1998) Neurogenesis in the adult human hippocampus. *Nature Medicine*, 4: 1313–1317.

Esteves, F. and Ohman, A. (1993) Masking the face: recognition of emotional facial expressions as a function of the parameters of backward masking. *Scandinavian Journal of Psychology*, 34: 1–18.

Eysenck, H.J. and Rachman, S.J. (1965) *Causes and Cures of Neurosis.* London: Routledge and Kegan Paul.

Fagan, B.F. (1998) *People of the Earth: an introduction to world prehistory.* New York: Longman.

Fanselow, M.S. (1980) Signalled shock-free periods and preference for signalled shock. *Journal of Experimental Psychology: Animal Behavior Processes*, 6: 65–80.

Favaro, A., Degortes, D., Colombo, G. and Santonastaso, P. (2000) The effects of trauma among kidnap victims in Sardinia, Italy. *Psychological Medicine*, 30: 975–980.

Fleming, P. (1995–1996) *Neanderthals.* Origins of Human Kind Research Center. http://www.pro-am.com/origins/research/neand3.htm

Fleshner, M., Laudenslager, M.L., Simons, L. and Maier, S.F. (1989) Reduced serum antibodies associated with social defeat in rats. *Physiology and Behavior*, 45: 1183–1187.

Foa, E.B. (1997) Trauma and women: course, predictors, and treatment. *Journal of Clinical Psychiatry*, 58: 25–28.

Foa, E.B. and Kozac, M.J. (1986) Emotional processing of fear: exposure to corrective information. *Psychological Bulletin*, 99: 20–35.

Foa, E.B., Zinbarg, R. and Rothbaum, B.O. (1992) Uncontrollability and unpredictability in posttraumatic stress disorder: an animal model. *Psychological Bulletin*, 112: 218–238.

Galea, S., Ahern, J., Resnick, H., Kilpatrick, D., Bucuvalas, M., Gold, J. and Vlahov, D. (2002a) Psychological sequelae of the September 11 terrorist attacks in New York City. *New England Journal of Medicine*, 346: 982–987.

Galea, S., Resnick, H., Ahern, J., Gold, J., Bucuvalas, M., Kilpatrick, D., Stuber, J. and Vlahov, D. (2002b) Posttraumatic stress disorder in Manhattan, New York City, after the September 11th terrorist attacks. *Journal of Urban Health*, 79(3): 340–353.

Galea, S., Vlahov, D., Resnick, H., Ahern, J., Susser, E., Gold, J., Bucuvalas, M. and Kilpatrick, D. (2003) Trends of probable posttraumatic stress disorder in New York City after the September 11 terrorist attacks. *American Journal of Epidemiology*, 158: 514–524.

Garcia, J., McGowan, B.K., Ervin, F.R. and Koelling, R.A. (1968) Cues: their relative effectiveness as a function of the reinforcer. *Science*, 160: 794–795.

Gardner, R. and Wilson, D.R. (2004) Sociophysiology and evolutionary aspects of psychiatry. In: *Textbook of Biological Psychiatry*. Ed: Panksepp, J. Hoboken, NJ: Wiley-Liss.

Geist, V. (1978) *Life Strategies, Human Evolution, Environmental Design.* New York: Springer Verlag.

Gilbert, P. (1992) *Depression: the evolution of powerlessness.* Hove: Lawrence Erlbaum.

Gilbert, P. (1993) Defence and safety: their function in social behaviour and psychopathology. *British Journal of Clinical Psychology*, 32: 131–153.

Gilbert, P. (1998) Evolutionary psychopathology: why isn't the mind designed better than it is? *British Journal of Medical Psychology*, 71: 353–373.

Gilbertson, M.W., Shenton, M.E., Ciszewski, A., Kasai, K., Lasko, N.B., Orr, S.P. and Pitman, R.K. (2002) Smaller hippocampal volume predicts pathological vulnerability to psychological trauma. *Nature and Neuroscience*, 5: 1242–1247.

Goddard, C.R. and Stanley, J.R. (1994) Viewing the abusive parent and the abused child as captor and hostage: the application of hostage theory to the effects of child abuse. *Journal of Interpersonal Violence*, 9: 258–269.

Gould, E., Beylin, A., Tanapat, P., Reeves, A. and Shors, T.J. (1999) Learning enhances adult neurogenesis in the hippocampal formation. *Nature Neuroscience*, 2: 260–265.

Graham, Y.P., Heim, C., Goodman, S.H., Miller, A.H. and Nemeroff, C.B. (1999) The effects of neonatal stress on brain development: implications for psychopathology. *Development and Psychopathology*, 11: 545–565.

Gray, J.A. (1982) *The Neuropsychology of Anxiety.* Oxford: Oxford University Press.

Gray, J.A. (1987) *The Psychology of Fear and Stress*, 2nd edn. Cambridge: Cambridge University Press.

Green, B.L. (1994) Psychosocial research in traumatic stress: an update. *Journal of Traumatic Stress*, 7: 341–362.

Green, B.L., Grace, M.C., Lindy, J.D., Gleser, G.C. and Leonard, A.C. (1990) Risk factors for PTSD and other diagnoses in the general sample of Vietnam veterans. *American Journal of Psychiatry*, 147: 729–733.

Greene, H.W. (1994) Antipredator mechanisms in reptiles. In: *Biology of the Reptilia: Volume 16, Ecology B.* Eds: Gans, C. and Huey, R.B. Ann Arbor, MI: Branta Books.

Greene, H.W. (1999) Natural history and behavioural homology. *Homology (Novartis Foundation Symposium 222)*, pp. 173–188. Chichester: Wiley.

Gross, D.R. (1992) *Discovering Anthropology.* Mountain View, CA: Mayfield.

Harlow, H.F. and Mears, C. (1979) *The Human Model: primate perspectives.* New York: John Wiley and Sons.

Herman, J.L. (1992) Complex PTSD: a syndrome in survivors of prolonged and repeated trauma. *Journal of Traumatic Stress*, 3: 377–391.

Hill, K. and Hurtado, A.M. (1989) Hunter-gatherers of the new world. *American Scientist*, 77: 437–443.

Horowitz, M.J. (1986) *Stress Response Syndromes.* New York: Jason Aronson.

Hueter, R.E., Murphy, C.J., Howland, M., Sivak, J.G., Paul-Murphy, J.R. and Howland, H.C. (2001) Refractive state and accommodation in the eyes of free-swimming versus restrained juvenile lemon sharks (*Negaprion brevirostris*). *Vision Research*, 41: 1885–1889.

Jackson, R.L., Alexander, J.H. and Maier, S.F. (1980) Learned helplessness, inactivity, and associative deficits: effects of inescapable shock on response choice escape learning. *Journal of Experimental Psychology: Animal Behavior Processes*, 6: 1–20.

Janoff-Bulman, R. and Frieze, I.H. (1983) A theoretical perspective for understanding reactions to victimization. *Journal of Social Issues*, 38: 1–17.

Joffe, J.M., Rawson, R.A. and Mulick, J.A. (1973) Control of their environment reduces emotionality in rats. *Science*, 180: 1383–1384.

Kardiner, A. (1941) *The Traumatic Neuroses of War. Psychosomatic Medicine Monograph II–III*. Menasha, WI: George Banta.

Kavaliers, M. and Choleris, E. (2001) Antipredator responses and defensive behavior: ecological and ethological approaches for the neurosciences. *Neuroscience and Biobehavioural Reviews*, 25: 577–586.

Keane, T.M., Zimering, R.T. and Caddell, J.M. (1985) A behavioural formulation of posttraumatic stress disorder in Vietnam veterans. *The Behavior Therapist*, 8: 9–12.

Kempermann, G. and Gage, F.H. (2002) New nerve cells for the adult brain. *Scientific American*, 12: 38–61.

Kendell, R. and Jablensky, A. (2003) Distinguishing between the validity and utility of psychiatric diagnoses. *American Journal of Psychiatry*, 160: 4–12.

Kilpatrick, D. and Resnick, H. (1992) PTSD associated with exposure to criminal victimization in clinical and community populations. In: *Posttraumatic Stress Disorder in Review: recent research and future directions*. Eds: Davidson, J. and Foa, E. Washington, DC: American Psychiatric Press.

Klein, L.C., Popke, E.J. and Grunberg, N.E. (1998) Sex differences in effects of opioid blockade on stress induced freezing behavior. *Pharmacology, Biochemistry and Behavior*, 68: 413–417.

Koch, M. (1999) The neurobiology of startle. *Progress in Neurobiology*, 59: 107–128.

Koenen, K.C. (2003) A brief introduction to genetic research in PTSD. *PTSD Research Quarterly*, 14: 1–2.

Krystal, J.H, Kosten, T.R., Southwick, S., Mason, J.W., Perry, B.D. and Giller, E.L. (1989) Neurobiological aspects of PTSD: review of clinical and preclinical studies. *Behavior Therapy*, 20: 177–198.

Kudryavtseva, N.N. (2000) Agonistic behavior: a model, experimental studies, and perspectives. *Neuroscience and Behavioural Physiology*, 30: 293–305.

Kuleshnyk, I. (1984) The Stockholm syndrome: towards an understanding. *Social Action and the Law*, 10: 37–42.

Kulka, R.A., Schlenger, W.E., Fairbank, J.A., Jordan, B.K., Hough, R.L., Marmar, C.R. and Weiss, D.S. (1990) *Trauma and the Vietnam War Generation: report of findings from the National Vietnam Veterans Readjustment Study*. New York: Brunner/Mazel.

Kummer, H. (1995) *In Quest of the Sacred Baboon*. Ewing, NJ: Princeton University Press.

Kushner, M.G., Riggs, D.S., Foa, E.B. and Miller, S.M. (1992) Perceived controllability and the development of posttraumatic stress disorder (PTSD) in crime victims. *Behavior Research and Therapy*, 31: 105–110.

Ladd, C., Owens, M. and Nemeroff, C. (1996) Persistent changes in corticotrophin-releasing factor neuronal systems induced by maternal deprivation. *Endocrinology*, 137: 1212–1218.

Lang, P.J., Davis, M. and Ohman, A. (2000) Fear and anxiety: animal models and human cognitive psychophysiology. *Journal of Affective Disorders*, 61: 137–159.

Laudenslager, M.L., Fleshner, M., Hofstadter, P., Held, P.E., Simons, L. and Maier, S.F. (1988) Suppression of specific antibody production by inescapable shock: stability under varying conditions. *Brain, Behavior and Immunity*, 2: 92–101.

Laufer, R.S., Frey-Wouters, E. and Gallops, M.S. (1985) Traumatic stressors in the Vietnam War and posttraumatic stress disorder. In: *Trauma and its Wake: the study and treatment of posttraumatic stress disorder*. Ed: Figley, C.R. New York: Brunner/Mazel.

LeDoux, J.E. (1996) *The Emotional Brain*. New York: Simon and Schuster.

LeDoux, J.E. (2002) Emotion, memory and the brain. *Scientific American*, 12: 62–71.

LeDoux, J.E. and Phelps, E.A. (2000) Emotional networks in the brain. In: *Handbook of Emotions*. Eds: Lewis, M. and Haviland-Jones, J.M. New York: Guilford.

LeDoux, J.E., Romanski, L. and Xagoraris, A. (1989) Indelibility of sub-cortical emotional memories. *Journal of Cognitive Neuroscience*, 1: 238–243.

Lee, D. and Turner, S. (1997) Theoretical models of posttraumatic stress disorder: cognitive-behavioural models of PTSD. In: *Psychological Trauma: a developmental approach*. Eds: Black, D., Newman, M., Harris-Hendriks, J. and Mezey, G. London: Gaskell.

Leite-Panissi, C.R. and Menescal-de-Oliveira, L. (2002) Central nucleus of the amygdala and the control of tonic immobility in guinea pigs. *Brain Research Bulletin*, 58: 13–19.

Lima, S.L. (1995) Collective detection of predatory attack by social foragers: fraught with ambiguity. *Animal Behavior*, 50: 1097–1108.

Lima, S.L. (1998) Stress and decision-making under the risk of predation:

recent developments from behavioural, reproductive and ecological perspectives. *Advances in the Study of Behavior*, 27: 215–290.

Lima, S.L. and Bednekoff, P.A. (1999a) Back to the basics of antipredatory vigilance: can nonvigilant animals detect attack? *Animal Behavior*, 58: 537–543.

Lima, S.L. and Bednekoff, P.A. (1999b) Temporal variation in danger drives antipredator behavior: the predation risk allocation hypothesis. *American Naturalist*, 153: 649–659.

Lima, S.L. and Dill, L.M. (1990) Behavioural decisions made under risk of predation: a review and prospectus. *Canadian Journal of Zoology*, 68: 619–640.

Litz, B.T. and Gray, M.J. (2002) Emotional numbing in posttraumatic stress disorder: current and future research directions. *Australian and New Zealand Journal of Psychiatry*, 36: 198–204.

Loftus, E.F., Loftus, G.R. and Messo, J. (1987) Some facts about 'Weapon Focus'. *Law and Human Behavior*, 11: 55–62.

Lovejoy, C.O. (1982) Models of human evolution. *Science*, 217: 304–305.

McCall, G.J. and Resick, P.A. (2003) A pilot study of PTSD symptoms among Kalahari Bushmen. *Journal of Traumatic Stress*, 16: 445–450.

McEwen, B.S. (2000) The neurobiology of stress: from serendipity to clinical relevance. *Brain Research Interactive*, 886: 172–189.

McFarlane, A.C. (1997) The prevalence and longitudinal course of PTSD: implications for the neurobiological models of PTSD. In: *Psychobiology of Posttraumatic Stress Disorder*. Eds: Yehuda, R. and McFarlane, A.C. New York: New York Academy of Sciences.

McFarlane, A.C. and De Girolamo, G. (1996) The nature of traumatic stressors and epidemiology of posttraumatic reactions. In: *Traumatic Stress: the effects of overwhelming experience on mind, body, and society*. Eds: van der Kolk, B.A., McFarlane, A.C. and Weisaeth, L. New York: Guilford.

McFarlane, A.C. and van der Kolk, B.A. (1996a) Trauma and its challenge to society. In: *Traumatic Stress: the effects of overwhelming experience on mind, body, and society*. Eds: van der Kolk, B.A., McFarlane, A.C. and Weisaeth, L. New York: Guilford.

McFarlane, A.C. and van der Kolk, B.A. (1996b) Conclusions and future directions. In: *Traumatic Stress: the effects of overwhelming experience on mind, body, and society*. Eds: van der Kolk, B.A., McFarlane, A.C. and Weisaeth, L. New York: Guilford.

McFarlane, A.C. and Yehuda, R. (1996) Resilience, vulnerability, and the course of posttraumatic reactions. In: *Traumatic Stress: the effects of overwhelming experience on mind, body, and society*. Eds: van der Kolk, B.A., McFarlane, A.C. and Weisaeth, L. New York: Guilford.

McGuire, M.T. and Triosi, A. (1998) *Darwinian Psychiatry*. New York: Oxford University Press.

McGuire, M.T., Marks, I., Nesse, R.M. and Triosi, A. (1992) Evolutionary biology: a basic science for psychiatry. *Acta Psychiatrica Scandanavica*, 86: 89–96.

MacLean, P.D. (1949) Psychosomatic disease and the 'visceral brain': recent developments bearing on the Papez theory of emotion. *Psychosomatic Medicine*, 11: 338–353.

MacLean, P.D. (1990) *The Triune Brain in Evolution: role in paleocerebral functions*. New York: Plenum Press.

MacLeod, A.D. (1994) The reactivation of posttraumatic stress disorder in later life. *Australian and New Zealand Journal of Psychiatry*, 28: 625–634.

Mariscano, G., Wotjak, C.T., Azad, S.C., Bisogno, T., Rammes, G., Cascio, M.G., et al. (2002) The endogenous cannabinoid system controls extinction of aversive memories. *Nature*, 418: 530–534.

Marks, I.M. (1987) *Fears, Phobias, and Rituals: panic, anxiety, and their disorders*. New York: Oxford University Press.

Marks, I.M. and Nesse, R.M. (1997) Fear and fitness: an evolutionary analysis of anxiety disorders. In: *The Maladapted Mind: classic readings in evolutionary psychology*. Ed: Baron-Cohen, S. Hove: Psychology Press.

Marshall, J.C., Halligan, P.W., Fink, G.R., Wade, D.T. and Frackowiak, R.S.J. (1997) The functional anatomy of a hysterical paralysis. *Cognition*, 64: B1–B8.

Mason, J.W., Wang, S., Yehuda, R., Riney, S., Charney, D.S. and Southwick, S.M. (2001) Psychogenic lowering of urinary cortisol levels linked to increased emotional numbing and a shame-depressive syndrome in combat-related posttraumatic stress disorder. *Psychosomatic Medicine*, 63: 387–401.

Maynard Smith, J. (1982) *Evolution and the Theory of Games*. Cambridge: Cambridge University Press.

Mayou, R., Bryant, B. and Duthie, R. (1993) Psychiatric consequences of road traffic accidents. *British Medical Journal*, 307: 647–651.

Mayr, E. (1974) Behavior programs and evolutionary strategies. *American Scientist*, 62: 650–659.

Mealey, L. (2000) *Sex Differences: developmental and evolutionary strategies*. San Diego, CA: Academic Press.

Miczec, K.A., Thompson, M.L. and Shuster, L. (1982) Opioid-like analgesia in defeated mice. *Science*, 215: 1520–1522.

Miller, L.E. (2002) An introduction to predator sensitive foraging. In: *Eat or Be Eaten: predator sensitive foraging among primates*. Ed: Miller, L.E. Cambridge: Cambridge University Press.

Mineka, S. (1987) A primate model of phobic fears. In: *Theoretical Foundations of Behaviour Therapy*. Eds: Eysenck, H. and Martin, I. New York: Plenum.

Mineka, S. (1992) Evolutionary memories, emotional processing, and the emotional disorders. In: *The Psychology of Learning and Motivation*, Volume 28. Ed: Medin, D. New York: Academic Press.

Mineka, S. and Cook, M. (1986) Immunization against observational conditioning of snake fear in rhesus monkeys. *Journal of Abnormal Psychology*, 95: 307–318.

Mineka, S. and Cook, M. (1993) Mechanisms involved in observational conditioning of fear. *Journal of Experimental Psychology: General*, 122: 23–38.

Mineka, S. and Hendersen, R.W. (1985) Controllability and predictability in acquired motivation. *Annual Reviews in Psychology*, 36: 495–529.

Mineka, S. and Zinbarg, R. (1991) Animal models of psychopathology. In: *Clinical Psychology: historical and research foundations*. Ed: Walker, C.E. New York and London: Plenum Press.

Mineka, S. and Zinbarg, R. (1995) Conditioning and ethological models of social phobia. In: *Social Phobia: diagnosis, assessment, and treatment*. Eds: Heimberg, R.G., Liebowitz, M.R., Hope, D.A. and Schneier, F.R. New York: Guilford.

Mineka, S., Gunnar, M. and Champoux, M. (1986) Control and early socio-emotional development: infant rhesus monkeys reared in controllable versus uncontrollable environments. *Child Development*, 57: 1241–1256.

Morris, J.S., Ohman, A. and Dolan, R.J. (1998) Conscious and unconscious emotional learning in the human amygdala. *Nature*, 393: 467–470.

Mowrer, O.H. and Viek, P. (1948) An experimental analogue of fear from a sense of helplessness. *Journal of Abnormal Psychology*, 43: 193–200.

Murray, J., Ehlers, A. and Mayou, R.A. (2002) Dissociation and post-traumatic stress disorder: two prospective studies of road traffic accident survivors. *British Journal of Psychiatry*, 180: 363–368.

Nategi, K. (1995–1996a) *Australopithecus (General)*. Origins of Human Kind Research Center. http://www.pro-am.com/origins/research/austgen1.htm

Nategi, K. (1995–1996b) *Homo habilis*. Origins of Human Kind Research Center. http://www.pro-am.com/origins/research/habilis1.htm

Nesse, R.M. (1997) An evolutionary perspective on panic disorder and agoraphobia. In: *The Maladapted Mind: classic readings in evolutionary psychology*. Ed: Baron-Cohen, S. Hove: Psychology Press.

Nesse, R.M. and Williams, G.C. (1998) Evolution and the origins of disease. *Scientific American*, November: 86–93.

Nijenhuis, E.R.S., Vanderlinden, J. and Spinhoven, P. (1998) Animal defence as a model for trauma-induced dissociative reactions. *Journal of Traumatic Stress*, 11: 243–260.

Nonacs, P. and Dill, L.M. (1990) Mortality risk vs. food quality in common currency: ant patch preferences. *Ecology*, 71: 1886–1892.

Norris, F.H. (1992) Epidemiology of trauma: frequency and impact of different potentially traumatic events on different demographic groups. *Journal of Consulting and Clinical Psychology*, 60: 409–418.

North, C.S., Nixon, S.J., Shariat, S., Mallonee, S., McMillen, J.C., Spitznagel, E.L. and Smith, E.M. (1999) Psychiatric disorders among survivors of the Oklahoma City bombing. *Journal of the American Medical Association*, 282: 755–762.

Ohman, A. (1986) Face the beast and face the fear: animal and social fears as prototypes for evolutionary analyses of emotion. *Psychophysiology*, 23: 123–145.

Ohman, A. and Mineka, S. (2001) Fears, phobias, and preparedness: toward an evolved module of fear and fear learning. *Psychological Review*, 108: 483–522.

Ohman, A. and Soares, J.J.F. (1994) 'Unconscious anxiety': phobic responses to masked stimuli. *Journal of Abnormal Psychology*, 103: 231–240.

Ohman, A., Dimberg, U. and Ost, L. (1985) Animal and social phobias: biological constraints on learned fear responses. In: *Theoretical issues in behavior therapy*. Eds: Reiss, S. and Bootzin, R.R. Orlando, FL: Academic Press.

Ohman, A., Flykt, A. and Lundqvist, D. (2000) Unconscious emotion: evolutionary perspectives, psychophysiological data, and neuropsychological mechanisms. In: *Cognitive Neuroscience of Emotion*. Eds: Lane, R.D. and Nadel, L. New York: Oxford University Press.

Overmier, J.B. and Seligman, M.E.P. (1967) Effects of inescapable shock upon subsequent escape and avoidance responding. *Journal of Comparative and Physiological Psychology*, 63: 28–33.

Panksepp, J. (1998) *Affective Neuroscience: the foundations of human and animal emotions*. New York: Oxford University Press.

Panksepp, J. (2000) Emotions as natural kinds within the mammalian brain. In: *Handbook of Emotions*. Eds: Lewis, M. and Haviland-Jones, J.M. New York: Guilford.

Parry-Jones, B. and Parry-Jones, W.L.L. (1994) Posttraumatic stress disorder: supportive evidence from an eighteenth century natural disaster. *Psychological Medicine*, 24: 15–27.

Pitman, R.K. and Orr, S. (1995) Psychophysiology of emotion and memory networks in posttraumatic stress disorder. In: *Brain and Memory: modulation and mediation of neuroplasticity*. Eds: Mcgaugh, J.L., Weinberger, N.M. and Lynch, G. New York: Oxford University Press.

Pitman, R.K., Orr, S.P., Forgue, D.F., Altman, B., de Jong, J.B. and Herz, L.R. (1990) Psychophysiologic responses to combat imagery of Vietnam veterans with posttraumatic stress disorder versus other anxiety disorders. *Journal of Abnormal Psychology*, 99: 49–54.

Plutchik, R. (1980) *Emotion: a psychoevolutionary synthesis*. New York: Harper and Row.

Potts, R. (1987) Reconstructions of early hominid socioecology: a critique of primate models. In: *The Evolution of Human Behavior: primate models*. Ed: Kinzey, W.G. Albany, NY: State University of New York Press.

Price, J. (1988) Alternative channels for negotiating asymmetry in social relationships. In: *Social Fabrics of the Mind*. Ed: Chance, M.R.A. Hove: Lawrence Erlbaum.

Price, J.S. and Sloman, L. (1987) Depression as yielding behavior: an animal model based on Schjelderup-Ebbe's pecking order. *Ethology and Sociobiology*, 8: 85S–98S.

Price, J.S., Gardner, R. and Erickson, M. (2004) Depression, anxiety and somatization as appeasement displays. *Journal of Affective Disorders*, 79: 1–11.

Proctor, C.J. and Broom, M. (2000) A spatial model of antipredator vigilance. *IMA Journal of Mathematics Applied in Medicine and Biology*, 17: 75–93.

Proctor, C.J., Broom, M. and Ruxton, G.D. (2001) Modelling antipredator vigilance and flight response in-group foragers when warning signals are ambiguous. *Journal of Theoretical Biology*, 211: 409–417.

Pynoos, R.S., Ritzmann, R.F., Steinberg, A.M. and Prisecaru, I. (1996) A behavioural animal model of posttraumatic stress disorder featuring repeated exposure to situational reminders. *Biological Psychiatry*, 39: 129–134.

Rakic, P. (2002) Neurogenesis in adult primate neocortex: an evaluation of the evidence. *Nature Reviews/Neuroscience*, 3: 65–71.

Ramos, A., Leite-Panissi, C., Monassi, C.R. and Menescal-de-Oliveira, L. (1999) Role of the amygdaloid nuclei in the modulation of tonic immobility in guinea pigs. *Physiology and Behavior*, 67: 717–724.

Remignon, H., Mills, A.D., Guemene, D., Desrosiers, V., Garreau-Mills, M. and Marche, M. (1998) Meat quality traits and muscle characteristics in high or low fear lines of Japanese quails (*Coturnix japonica*) subjected to acute stress. *British Poultry Science*, 39: 372–378.

Resnick, H.S., Yehuda, R., Pitman, R.K. and Foy, D.W. (1995) Effect of previous trauma on acute plasma cortisol level following rape. *American Journal of Psychiatry*, 152: 1675–1677.

Ridley, M. (1994) *The Red Queen: sex and the evolution of human nature*. London: Penguin.

Roth, S., Newman, E., Pelcovitz, D., van der Kolk, B. and Mandel, F.S. (1997) Complex PTSD in victims exposed to sexual and physical abuse: results from the DSM-IV field trial for posttraumatic stress disorder. *Journal of Traumatic Stress*, 10: 539–555.

Rothbaum, B.O., Meadows, E.A., Resick, P. and Foy, D.W. (2000) Cognitive behaviour therapy. In: *Effective Treatments for PTSD*. Eds: Foa, E.B., Keane, T.M. and Friedman, M.J. New York: Guilford.

Ruscio, A.M., Ruscio, J. and Keane, T.M. (2002) The latent structure of posttraumatic stress disorder: a taxometric investigation of reactions to extreme stress. *Journal of Abnormal Psychology*, 111: 290–301.

Sadock, B.J. and Sadock, V.A. (2000) *Kaplan and Sadock's Comprehensive*

Textbook of Psychiatry, 7th edn. Philadelphia, PA: Lippincott Williams and Wilkins.

Sauther, M.L. (2002) Group size effects on predation sensitive foraging in wild ring-tailed lemurs (*Lemur catta*). In: *Eat or Be Eaten: predator sensitive foraging among primates*. Ed: Miller, L.E. Cambridge: Cambridge University Press.

Schelde, T. and Hertz, M. (1994) Ethology and psychotherapy. *Ethology and Sociobiology*, 15: 383–392.

Scott, J.P. (1977) Agonistic behavior: function and dysfunction in social conflict. *Journal of Social Issues*, 33: 9–21.

Scott, J.P. and Marston, M. (1953) Nonadaptive behavior resulting from a series of defeats in fighting mice. *Journal of Abnormal and Social Psychology*, 48: 417–428.

Scurfield, R.M. (1985) Traumatic stressors in the Vietnam War and posttraumatic stress disorder. In: *Trauma and its Wake: the study and treatment of posttraumatic stress disorder*. Ed: Figley, C.R. New York: Brunner/Mazel.

Searleman, A. and Herrman, D. (1994) Effects of arousal, stress and emotion. In: *Memory from a Broader Perspective*. Eds: Searleman, A. and Herrman, D. New York: McGraw-Hill.

Seligman, M.E.P. (1971) Phobias and preparedness. *Behavior Therapy*, 2: 307–320.

Seligman, M.E.P. (1975) *Helplessness: on depression development and death*. San Francisco, CA: Freeman.

Seligman, M.E.P. and Maier, S.F. (1967) Failiure to escape traumatic shock. *Journal of Experimental Psychology*, 74: 1–9.

Setiawan, E., Knott, C.D. and Budhi, S. (1996) Preliminary assessment of vigilance and predator avoidance behavior of orangutans in Gunung Palung national park, West Kalimantan, Indonesia. *Tropical Diversity*, 3: 269–279.

Shalev, A.Y. (1996) Stress versus traumatic stress: from homeostatic reactions to chronic psychopathology. In: *Traumatic Stress: the effects of overwhelming experience on mind, body, and society*. Eds: van der Kolk, B.A., McFarlane, A.C. and Weisaeth, L. New York: Guilford.

Shapiro, F. (1999) Eye movement desensitization and reprocessing (EMDR) and the anxiety disorders: clinical and research implications of an integrated psychotherapy treatment. *Journal of Anxiety Disorders*, 13: 35–67.

Shephard, B. (2002) *A War of Nerves: soldiers and psychiatrists 1914–1994*. London: Pimlico.

Shorter, E. (1986) Paralysis – the rise and fall of a hysterical symptom. *Journal of Social History* 19: 549–582.

Sih, A. (1990) Prey uncertainty and the balancing of antipredator and feeding needs. *American Naturalist*, 139: 1052–1069.

Sih, A. (1992) Integrative approaches to the study of predation: general thoughts and a case study on sunfish and salamander larvae. *Annales Zoologici Fennici*, 29: 183–198.

Silove, D. (1998) Is posttraumatic stress disorder an overlearned survival response? An evolutionary-learning hypothesis. *Psychiatry*, 61: 181–190.

Solomon, Z., Laor, N. and McFarlane, A.C. (1996) Acute posttraumatic reactions in soldiers and civilians. In: *Traumatic Stress: the effects of overwhelming experience on mind, body, and society*. Eds: van der Kolk, B.A., McFarlane, A.C. and Weisaeth, L. New York: Guilford.

Spiegel, D., Hunt, T. and Dondershine, H.E. (1988) Dissociation and hypnotisability in posttraumatic stress disorder. *American Journal of Psychiatry*, 145: 301–305.

Staner, L. (2003) Sleep and anxiety disorders. *Dialogues in Clinical Neuroscience*, 5: 249–258.

Stanford, C.B. (1998) *Chimpanzee and Red Colobus: the ecology of predator and prey*. Cambridge, MA: Harvard University Press.

Stearns, S.C. and Hoekstra, R.F. (2000) *Evolution: an introduction*. Oxford: Oxford University Press.

Stein, D.J. (1998) Introduction: steps toward a comparative clinical psychopharmacology. In: *Psychopharmacology of Animal Behavior Disorders*. Eds: Dodman, N.H. and Shuster, L. Malden, MA: Blackwell Science.

Stevens, A. and Price, J. (1996) *Evolutionary Psychiatry: a new beginning*. London: Routledge.

Strentz, T. (1979) The Stockholm syndrome: law enforcement policy and ego defences of the hostage. *Annals of the New York Academy of Sciences*, 347: 137–150.

Strum, S.C. and Mitchell, W. (1987) Baboons: baboon models and muddles. In: *The Evolution of Human Behavior: primate models*. Ed: Kinzey, W.G. Albany, NY: State University of New York Press.

Suomi, S.J. (1991) Adolescent depression and depressive symptoms: insights from longitudinal studies with rhesus monkeys. *Journal of Youth and Adolescence* 20: 273–287.

Susman, R. (1987) Pygmy chimpanzees and common chimpanzees: models for behavioural ecology of the earliest hominids. In: *The Evolution of Human Behavior: primate models*. Ed: Kinzey, W.G. Albany, NY: State University of New York Press.

Tanapat, P., Hastings, N.B., Rydel, T.A., Galea, L.A.M. and Gould, E. (2001) Exposure to fox odor inhibits cell proliferation in the hippocampus of adult rats via an adrenal hormone dependent mechanism. *Journal of Comparative Neurology*, 437: 496–504.

Tanner, N.M. (1987) Gathering by females: the chimpanzee model revisited and the gathering hypothesis. In: *The Evolution of Human Behavior: primate models*. Ed: Kinzey, W.G. Albany, NY: State University of New York Press.

Tennant, C. (2004) Psychological trauma: psychiatry and the law in conflict. *Australian and New Zealand Journal of Psychiatry*, 38: 344–347.

Thompson, S.B. (1998) Pharmacologic treatment of phobias. In: *Psychopharmacology of animal behavior disorders*. Eds: Dodman, N.H. and Shuster, L. Malden, MA: Blackwell Science.

Tooby, J. and Cosmides, L. (1990) The past explains the present: emotional adaptations and the structure of ancestral environments. *Ethology and Sociobiology*, 11: 375–424.

Tooby, J. and Cosmides, L. (2000) Evolutionary psychology and the emotions. In: *Handbook of Emotions*. Eds: Lewis, M. and Haviland-Jones, J.M. New York: Guilford.

Toth, S.L. and Cicchetti, D. (1998) Remembering, forgetting, and the effects of trauma on memory: a developmental psychology perspective. *Development and Psychopathology*, 10: 589–605.

Treves, A. (1998) Primate social systems: conspecific threat and coercion-defense hypotheses. *Folia Primatology*, 69: 81–88.

Treves, A. (2000) Theory and method in studies of vigilance and aggregation. *Animal Behaviour*, 60: 711–722.

Treves, A. (2002) Predicting predation risk for foraging, arboreal monkeys. In: *Eat or Be Eaten: predator sensitive foraging in non-human primates*. Ed: Miller, L. Cambridge: Cambridge University Press.

Treves, A. (in preparation) Reconstructing the antipredator behavior of early hominids.

Treves, A. and Pizzagalli, D. (2002) Vigilance and perception of social stimuli: views from ethology and social neuroscience. In: *The Cognitive Animal: empirical and theoretical perspectives on animal cognition*. Eds: Bekoff, M., Allen, C. and Burghardt, G.M. Cambridge, MA: MIT Press.

Trivers, R. (1985) *Social Evolution*. Menlo Park, CA: Benjamin/Cummings.

True, W.R., Rice, J., Eisen, S.A., Heath, A.C., Goldberg, J., Lyons, M.J. and Nowak, J. (1993) A twin study of genetic and environmental contributions to liability for posttraumatic stress symptoms. *Archives of General Psychiatry*, 50: 257–264.

Tsuang, M.T., Bar, J.L., Stone, W.S. and Faraone, S.V. (2004) Gene environment interaction in mental disorders. *World Psychiatry*, 3: 73–83.

Tsukahara, T. (1993) Lions eat chimpanzees: the first evidence of predation by lions on wild chimpanzees. *American Journal of Primatology*, 29: 1–11.

Turco, R.M. (1987) Psychiatric contributions to the understanding of international terrorism. *International Journal of Offender Therapy and Comparative Criminology*, 31: 153–161.

Valentiner, D.P., Foa, E.B., Riggs, D.S. and Gershuny, B.S. (1996) Coping strategies and posttraumatic stress disorder in female victims of sexual and nonsexual assault. *Journal of Abnormal Psychology*, 3: 455–458.

van der Kolk, B.A. (1987) *Psychological Trauma*. Washington, DC: American Psychiatric Press.

van der Kolk, B.A. (1989) The compulsion to re-enact the trauma: re-enactment, re-victimisation and masochism. *Psychiatric Clinics of North America*, 12: 389–411.

van der Kolk, B.A. (1994) The body keeps the score: memory and the evolving psychobiology of posttraumatic stress disorder. *Harvard Review of Psychiatry*, 1: 253–265.

van der Kolk, B.A. (1996a) The complexity of adaptation to trauma: self-regulation, stimulus discrimination, and characterological development. In: *Traumatic Stress: the effects of overwhelming experience on mind, body, and society*. Eds: van der Kolk, B.A., McFarlane, A.C. and Weisaeth, L. New York: Guilford.

van der Kolk, B.A. (1996b) Trauma and memory. In: *Traumatic Stress: the effects of overwhelming experience on mind, body, and society*. Eds: van der Kolk, B.A., McFarlane, A.C. and Weisaeth, L. New York: Guilford.

van der Kolk, B.A. (1996c) The body keeps the score: approaches to the psychobiology of posttraumatic stress disorder. In: *Traumatic Stress: the effects of overwhelming experience on mind, body, and society*. Eds: van der Kolk, B.A., McFarlane, A.C. and Weisaeth, L. New York: Guilford.

van der Kolk, B.A. and McFarlane, A.C. (1996) The black hole of trauma. In: *Traumatic Stress: the effects of overwhelming experience on mind, body, and society*. Eds: van der Kolk, B.A., McFarlane, A.C. and Weisaeth, L. New York: Guilford.

van der Kolk, B., van der Hart, O. and Marmar, C.R. (1996a) Dissociation and information processing in posttraumatic stress disorder. In: *Traumatic Stress: the effects of overwhelming experience on mind, body, and society*. Eds: van der Kolk, B.A., McFarlane, A.C. and Weisaeth, L. New York: Guilford.

van der Kolk, B.A., Weisaeth, L. and van der Hart, O. (1996b) History of trauma in psychiatry. In: *Traumatic Stress: the effects of overwhelming experience on mind, body, and society*. Eds: van der Kolk, B.A., McFarlane, A.C. and Weisaeth, L. New York: Guilford.

van Praag, H.M. (2004) Stress and suicide: are we well-equipped to study this issue? *Crisis*, 25: 80–85.

van Praag, H., Schinder, A.F., Christie, B.R., Toni, N., Palmer, T.D. and Gage, F.H. (2002) Functional neurogenesis in the adult hippocampus. *Nature*, 415: 1030–1034.

Vermeij, G.J. (1982) Unsuccessful predation and evolution. *The American Naturalist*, 120: 701–720.

Walker, E.L. (1958) Action decrement and its relation to learning. *Psychological Review*, 65: 129–142.

Watts, D.P. (1998) A preliminary study of selective visual attention in female mountain gorillas (*Gorilla gorilla berengei*). *Primates*, 39: 71–78.

Weed, S. (1976) *My Search for Patty Hearst*. London: Secker and Warburg.

Wenegrat, B. (1984) *Sociobiology and Mental Disorder: a new view.* Menlo Park, CA: Addison-Wesley.

West, L.J. and Martin, P.R. (1994) Pseudo-identity and the treatment of personality change in victims of captivity and cults. In: *Dissociation: clinical and theoretical perspectives.* Eds: Lynn, S.J. and Rhue, J.W. New York: Guilford.

Williams, G.C. and Nesse, R.M. (1991) The dawn of Darwinian medicine. *Quarterly Review of Biology,* 66: 1–22.

Williams, J. and Lierle, D.M. (1988) Effects of repeated defeat by a dominant conspecific on subsequent pain sensitivity, open-field activity, and escape learning. *Animal Learning and Behavior,* 16: 477–485.

Wilson, M.A. and McNaughton, B.L. (1994) Reactivation of hippocampal ensemble memories during sleep. *Science,* 265: 676–679.

Wirtz, P. and Wawra, M. (1986) Vigilance and group size in Homo sapiens. *Ethology,* 71: 283–286.

World Health Organization (1992) *International Statistical Classification of Diseases and Related Health Problems,* 10th edn, volume 1. Geneva: World Health Organization.

Wortman, C.B. and Brehm, J.W. (1975) Responses to uncontrollable outcomes. An integration of reactance theory and the learned helplessness model. In: *Advances in Experimental Social Psychology,* Volume 8. New York: Academic Press.

Wrangham, R.W. (1979) On the evolution of ape social systems. *Social Science Information,* 18: 335–368.

Wrangham, R.W. (1986) Ecology and social relationships in two species of chimpanzee. In: *Ecology and Social Evolution: birds and mammals.* Eds: Rubenstein, I. and Wrangham, R.W. Princeton, NJ: Princeton University Press.

Wrangham, R.W. (1999a) Evolution of coalitionary killing. *Yearbook of Physical Anthropology,* 42: 1–30.

Wrangham, R.W. (1999b) Is military incompetence adaptive? *Evolution and Human Behavior* 20: 3–17.

Wrangham, R. and Peterson D. (1996) *Demonic Males: apes and the origins of human violence.* London: Bloomsbury.

Yehuda, R. (1999) Linking the neuroendocrinology of posttraumatic stress disorder with recent neuroanatomic findings. *Seminars in Clinical Neuropsychiatry,* 4: 256–265.

Yehuda, R. and McFarlane, A.C. (1995) Conflict between current knowledge about posttraumatic stress disorder and its original conceptual basis. *American Journal of Psychiatry,* 152: 1705–1713.

Yehuda, R., McFarlane, A.C. and Shalev, A.Y. (1998) Predicting the development of posttraumatic stress disorder from the acute response to a traumatic event. *Biological Psychiatry,* 44: 1305–1313.

Yerkes, R.M. and Dodson, J.D. (1908) The relation of strength of stimulus to rapididty of habit-formation. *Journal of Comparative Neurology and Psychology*, 18: 459–482.

Zlotnick, C., Warshaw, M., Shea, M.T., Allsworth, J., Pearlstein, T. and Keller, M.B. (1999) Chronicity in posttraumatic stress disorder (PTSD) and predictors of course of comorbid PTSD in patients with anxiety disorders. *Journal of Traumatic Stress*, 12: 89–100.

Zulkifli, I., Che-Norma, M.T., Chong, C.H. and Loh, T.C. (2000) Heterophil to lymphocyte ratio and tonic immobility reactions to pre-slaughter handling in broiler chickens treated with ascorbic acid. *Poultry Science*, 79: 402–406.

Index